AF597384

THE ROLE OF HOSPITALS IN GERIATRIC CARE

The Role of Hospitals in Geriatric Care

Carl Eisdorfer, Ph.D., M.D.
George L. Maddox, Ph.D.
Editors

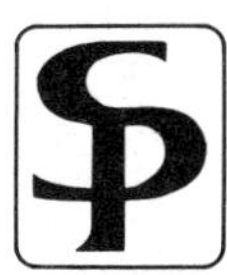

SPRINGER PUBLISHING COMPANY
New York

Springer Publishing Company, Inc.
536 Broadway
New York, NY 10012

88 89 90 91 92 / 5 4 3 2 1

LIBRARY OF CONGRESS
Library of Congress Cataloging-in-Publication Data

The Role of hospitals in geriatric care / Carl Eisdorfer, George L. Maddox, editors.
p. cm.
Papers presented at the XIIIth Congress of IAG, held in New York in 1985.
Includes bibliographies and index.
ISBN 0-8261-5310-0
1. Aged—Hospital care. I. Eisdorfer, Carl. II. Maddox, George L. III. International Congress of Gerontology (13th : 1985 : New York, N.Y.)
[DNLM: 1. Delivery of Health Care—congresses. 2. Geriatrics—congresses. 3. Health Services for the Aged—congresses. 4. Hospitals—congresses. WT 30 R745 1985]
RC954.3.R65 1988
362.1.'9897—dc19
DNLM/DLC
for Library of Congress 87-35625
CIP

Printed in the United States of America

Contents

Preface

In 1950, the International Association of Gerontology (IAG) was chartered as a multidisciplinary organization to facilitate the worldwide exchange of information about research, education, and practice related to human aging. Periodic congresses facilitate this exchange. The XIIIth and most recent congress of the IAG was held in New York in 1985.

Among the symposia recommended for development by the planning committee was a critical discussion of the role of the hospital in the continuum of geriatric care. Is there a distinctive role for the hospital and, if so, what is that role? The stimulus for asking these questions was the considerable evidence of ambivalence and conflicting opinions in the United States about the relative contributions of formal systems of geriatric medical care concentrated in hospitals in contrast to a broader range of health care systems in the community. An international meeting seemed to be an appropriate place to explore whether professionals from other developed societies with a variety of cultural perspectives understood the question as asked by professionals in the United States and if they found the subject interesting. Perspectives from Canada, Israel, Sweden, and the United Kingdom were presented in the discussion. The multidisciplinary international meeting provided further opportunity to examine how such questions are explored and answered by physicians, nurses, health administrators, and an assortment of persons trained variously in law, social work, political science, sociology, psychology, and policy analysis.

With the encouragement and partial financial support of the

Robert Wood Johnson Foundation, Carl Eisdorfer and George Maddox initially asked four colleagues to develop position papers addressing the question, "Is there a distinctive role for the hospital in the continuum of care for the elderly, and, if so, what is that role?" These papers, which appear as Chapters 2 to 5 in this volume, were the response. Whether and how well these questions were addressed is for the reader to decide; but the evidence of obvious difficulty in providing a consensual answer is, in part, a measure of the problem that prompted the symposium in the first place.

These four position papers were circulated well in advance of the Congress, and a number of discussants reacted critically. These reactions are recorded as Chapters 6 to 10 in this volume. The authors of the position papers and their critics met prior to the Congress for a day-long discussion and then shared a distillation of their agreements and disagreements at the Congress in a formal presentation of a symposium to a standing-room-only audience of 250. In the months following the Congress, the initial authors and their critics sharpened their statements, and this book is the outcome.

Readers of this volume may also be interested in two other volumes recording the work of the XIIIth Congress of IAG, both published by Springer Publishing Company in 1987. The first is *Aging: The Universal Human Experience,* edited by George Maddox and E. W. Busse, which records highlights from a broad multidisciplinary and cross-national range of symposia on biological, medical, behavioral, social-scientific, and social policy aspects of human aging. The second is *Epidemiology and Aging,* edited by Jacob Brody and George Maddox, which illustrates the uses of epidemiology worldwide to describe the age-related distribution of health and disease, reports new information on the epidemiology of mental health and illness, and shows how epidemiological information can be usefully applied to program planning and policy development in aging societies.

We thank our colleagues who made possible the symposium and this presentation of their views on geriatric health care.

CARL EISDORFER AND GEORGE MADDOX
July, 1987

Editors and Contributors

Editors

Carl Eisdorfer, Ph.D., M.D., is chairman of the Department of Psychiatry and Director of the Center for Aging, University of Miami. His career in academic psychological and biomedical research has been complemented by experience as the chief executive officer of a major medical center and hospital.

George L. Maddox, Ph.D., is professor of sociology and chairman of the University Council on Aging and Human Development, Duke University. He is Secretary General of the International Association of Gerontology.

Contributors

Stanley J. Brody, J.D., M.S.W., is professor of physical medicine and rehabilitation in psychiatry, Department of Physical Medicine and Rehabilitation, and Director, Research and Training Center for Rehabilitation of Elderly Disabled Individuals, University of Pennsylvania.

Miriam J. Hirschfeld, R.N., D.N.Sc., is a Senior Lecturer in the Department of Nursing, Tel-Aviv University, and National Coordinator for Care of the Aged, Kupat Holim, Health Insurance Institute of the General Federation of Labour, Israel.

Robert L. Kane, M.D., is Dean of the School of Public Health, University of Minnesota at Minneapolis. Previously he was professor of geriatric medicine at the University of California at Los Angeles and a Senior Investigator at the Rand Corporation, Santa Monica. His work has focused on evaluation of long-term care.

Mathy D. Mezey, R.N., Ed.D., F.A.A.N., is Director of the Teaching Nursing Home Program, School of Nursing, University of Pennsylvania. She is coordinator of the Robert Wood Johnson Foundation Program on the Teaching Nursing Home.

Anne R. Somers is Adjunct Professor, Rutgers Medical School, University of Medicine and Dentistry of New Jersey. She is a well-known proponent of preventive and innovative geriatric care.

Alvar Svanborg, M.D., Ph.D., is Professor of Geriatric Medicine in the Department of Geriatric and Long-Term Care Medicine, Vasa Hospital, University of Göteborg, Sweden. He is an advisor to the Swedish National Board of Health and Welfare and to the World Health Organization. He is currently President of the Federation of Gerontology of the Nordic countries.

Malcolm G. Taylor, Ph.D., LL.D., is Emeritus Professor of Public Policy at York University, Toronto, Canada. He has served as research consultant to the Royal Commission on Health Services (1961–1964) and the Health Services Review (1979–1980).

Bruce C. Vladeck, Ph.D., is President of the United Hospital Fund of New York, the nation's oldest federated charity. Educated at Harvard and the University of Michigan, he has been actively involved in the development of prospective payment systems in health care and critical evaluation of long-term care policy in the United States.

James Williamson, CBE, MB, FRCPE, is Professor Emeritus, Geriatric Medicine, University of Edinburgh, Scotland. He has served as President of the British Geriatrics Society.

THE ROLE OF HOSPITALS IN GERIATRIC CARE

1
A Distinctive Role for Hospitals in Caring for Older Adults: Issues and Options

Carl Eisdorfer and George Maddox

In recent decades, hospitals have played a dominant role in providing health care for older adults. In the United States in 1985, the elderly accounted for more than a third of all inpatient days of hospital care (approximately 96 million bed days, or 40%) and for 36 million hospital outpatient visits. Older adults on average spent three times more days in hospitals than did adults generally, and this pattern has been relatively consistent since the early days of the financing of Medicare. It has been estimated that approximately 70% of Medicare health care dollars have been expended on the provision of hospital-based services, thus making hospitals that serve older adults the major economic beneficiaries among the various health care providers. Will this dominance of hospitals in geriatric care continue? Probably yes, but there is evidence of change in the wind. (For a succinct review of current evidence regarding the hospitalization and long-term care of older adults, see Rabin and Stockton, 1987.)

INTENT OF MEDICARE

Data documenting the centrality of hospitals in geriatric care clearly reflect the intent of the original Medicare legislation. That intent had predictable effects on ensuring a dominant role of hospitals in geriatric care. In the early 1960s, U.S. health and social policy was dedicated to providing access for older adults to the same type of health insurance coverage that was already available to most of the adult population through employment-related benefit programs. The expenses of surgery and hospitalization in particular were the most costly burdens being faced by older persons, and by their children as well; covering the costs of these most expensive components of care was the primary objective of Medicare legislation. Medicare was, and remains, primarily a form of social insurance to offset the cost of care for acute illness and surgery—paralleling the programs offered by private health insurance for employed younger and middle-aged adults. Early in the development of Medicare, restrictions were placed on the nature of the reimbursement formulae as a way to deal politically with the criticism that the program would lead to socialized medicine in the United States and impair the doctor–patient relationship. As a consequence, policy at that time was intended to minimize the impact of Medicare on the existing fee-for-service practice of medicine. Medicare also followed initially the practices of insurance companies in reimbursing hospitals on a fee-for-service basis for inpatient care. Long-term care, it should be noted, was specifically deemphasized in the Medicare legislation. Medicare, the principle resource for the funding of health care for the elderly, was thus developed as a mechanism primarily for the funding of acute care; its bias was toward inpatient acute care, away from long-term care, and calculated not to challenge the existing fee-for-service payment system.

MEDICARE'S IMPACT

Since its inception in 1965, Medicare has provided a significant degree of assistance for acute medical and surgical care to many older Americans. Before Medicare, 68% of the elderly saw a physician at least annually. Approximately 20 years later, 93% of the elderly could identify a regular source of medical care. The vast majority of elderly, including the elderly poor, can now identify a private doctor or clinic that they use instead of hospital outpatient clinics or emergency rooms, which were common sources of care pre-Medicare. Prior to Medicare, the poor used hospitals less than the nonpoor, but today that situation is reversed; and the gap between the poor and nonpoor in the use of physician services has also been eliminated. Indeed, the increase in the amount and intensity of services suggested by more equal access of poor and nonpoor persons accounts for about one third of the annual increase in health care costs. Thus, the original objective of the Medicare legislation, to serve the underserved elderly, seems to have been substantially achieved.

Although it is not possible to assess directly the relationship between health outcome and Medicare's success in improving access to health care, it is clear that mortality has declined continuously since the establishment of Medicare; and gains in longevity for nonwhites and the poor (those who seemed to have profited most from the availability of Medicare) have been greater than the gains for whites. This, at least in part, may be attributable to the increased utilization of Medicare-supported health care.

The amount and distribution of health dollars has changed significantly. In 1965, total health care expenditures for the aged were $8.9 billion, with approximately 30% financed out of public funds. By 1978, however, public programs were financing 87.5% of hospital expenditures and 46.2% of nursing home costs for the elderly.

The cost of geriatric care is high. Because this cost is substantially related to the primacy of the hospital's role in caring for older persons, interest in alternatives to hospital care persists. Some experienced observers do wonder whether hospitalization is the most appropriate way to meet many of the health care needs of older persons. It is sometimes difficult to know whether complaints about hospital care for older adults stem from an assessment of poor or inappropriate care, or from its cost. Attacking hospital care can be merely a screen to divert attention from other less socially attractive concerns, such as reducing expenditures on older patients or the competition among health care organizations for scarce funds. In an effort to clarify the issues, first let us examine briefly some basic issues in hospital care costs.

FACTORS IN HOSPITAL CARE COST

For a variety of reasons, in recent decades hospital care has become progressively more expensive. In part, higher cost is the result of substantial improvements in health care technology and related substantial increases in capital costs. Thus, in diagnostic radiology the transition from x-rays to CT scans to Magnetic Resonance Imaging (MRIs) has led to increases in capital costs and the cost of care. Additionally, interest charges on money borrowed to pay for such equipment and the need for technicians with sophisticated training have produced higher operating costs. Although such costs obviously lend themselves to documentation relatively easily, the clinical value of any improvement over the preceding technology is sustantially harder to document. For example, the dollars expended on major joint surgery are simple to determine, but the resultant improvements in quality of life for older persons with hip replacement, as well as the impact on their families, appear to be too subjective to put into any simple econometric model.

The cost of hospital-based biomedical technology is only one of the issues in the increase of the expense of care. The cost of hospital-based personnel has risen for a variety of reasons. These include the improvement of employee salaries and benefits resulting from collective bargaining; investment in better-trained and therefore higher-salaried technicians, nurses, and others to deal with more sophisticated equipment and procedures; a larger spectrum of personnel than had been previously employed; and increasingly sicker patients in hospitals with the concomitant increase in the intensity of care. In addition, the cost of administration and the bureaucracy required by third-party payers has itself become a significant economic burden for hospitals. Because cost of care is more readily measured than are outcomes of care, the focus on the negative aspect of the equation—with great attention to the cost and relatively little to quality of care—is a likely outcome.

The use of hospital beds in lieu of other types of care did increase for a time following enactment of Medicare legislation. In view of the fact that hospital care was reimbursable whereas most other forms of care were not, this is not surprising. The longstanding pattern of reimbursing hospitals on what was essentially a cost-plus basis only reinforced the tendency toward longer length of stays without regard for the cost involved. Indeed, for decades increased hospitalization was driven, in part, by insurance reimbursement for expensive laboratory tests provided on an inpatient basis only.

PHYSICIANS AND HEALTH COSTS

Traditionally, physicians have played a dominant role in deciding on the need for a patient's hospitalization without themselves having responsibility for any of the cost incurred. Economists refer to the physicians as "secondary demand" because, once patients place themselves under the management of physicians, the physicians make the specific decisions that generate health care costs. Because physicians, at least in the United States, are assumed to be the agents of their patients and to pursue their interests primarily if not exclusively, physicians in private practice have had little economic incentive to minimize the cost of care. Indeed, they have had some incentive to practice defensive medicine to protect against malpractice suits by performing more tests and procedures on the patient than would be required by medical considerations alone.

HEALTH AS A VALUE

Americans value health, and they associate health care with physicians, high technology, and hospitals. Note, for example, the great disparity between the availability of funds to pay for medical care as opposed to other human services, particularly for older Americans. These values and related responses have led to an exaggerated and inappropriate medicalization of many of the problems of older persons. This simplification is unfortunate because biological, psychological, and social variables interact distinctively in later life so that functional impairments and disabilities are not typically biological, or psychological, or social, but are a mixture of all three. This point has been noted by the health and welfare professionals who provide formal care for older adults. But these professionals have found it difficult to translate their insights into appropriate organizational responses. Some hospitals, for example, have tended to develop a social component of care; and currently many hospitals are exploring new ways of organizing care vertically and horizontally in order to supply a wide range of services to the community and to reach people not typically associated with the community hospital. The expanded role of hospitals has not, however, routinely proved to be economical or demonstrably effective in providing better geriatric care.

Health care costs have increased, in part, as a result of inefficiency in the ways hospitals deliver care. Too many hospitals want to own and operate high-cost technology on an independent basis; and too many want to fund expensive programs (e.g., cardiac surgery) in competition with neighboring hospitals, even when the aggregated patient needs in the community do not warrant such duplication of service. Focusing on high technology and spectacular cures is encouraged by the complementary interests of industry, hospitals, and health care personnel. Health care providers are well aware there is a large market for health services, and they are willing to use media promotion of high-technology medicine to increase their share of that market. Older adults have proved to be a very good market. Since the enactment of Medicare, older adults have become principal users of the services of physicians and hospitals. Older persons, who constitute about 11% of the population, consume health services at a rate two to three times higher than do adults generally. The average physician can expect 30% of the patients served to be older adults, and the average community hospital has become a geriatric institution.

A CHANGE IN THE WIND

For older adults, hospitalization is often a mixed blessing. Long stays in hospitals for older patients may lead to secondary medical consequences, for example, hospital-based infections or decubiti, and decreased capacity of the older patient to function in any community to which they might be returned following hospitalization. The advent of the diagnostic-related (DRG) reimbursement mechanism for Medicare patients has provided an occasion for hospitals and physicians to review current practices with an interest in reducing days in hospital. The emphasis now is on minimizing rather than maximizing hospital use and reducing length of stay—and length of hospital stays among older adults has in fact been decreasing. But the new reimbursement system has generated complaints from some health care advocates that older patients are being discharged from hospital care "quicker and sicker," and that we are creating a new set of health problems for older adults, particularly in the absence of an organized network of community-based care. One rarely encounters the argument that shorter stays in hospitals might be, on average, good for older patients, particularly if they are discharged into a community with an adequate array of supportive services.

THE FUTURE OF GERIATRIC HEALTH CARE

A substantial debate about the appropriate roles of the hospital in a community, particularly in regard to care of the aged, has therefore emerged. This debate was the occasion for the symposium whose papers are collected here. There are a number of options to consider as the future role of hospitals in the care of older adults is discussed. Two major options are obvious.

Hospitals can be conceived as extended emergency service providers, very much on the order of a police or fire station. In this conception, it is appropriate to have a high-technology setting and qualified staff who are adequately supported to await emergencies. In response to medical emergencies, they play out their relatively brief but intense and socially important role. At an extreme, this model is already observed in communities with emergency and trauma networks, where hospital emergency rooms are organized to receive patients by levels of disability on the basis of geographically defined service areas. Victims needing emergency care are transported to the nearest hospital with appropriate services. Even nonemergency but certain acutely needed or scheduled care (e.g., kidney transplant, or the diagnosis and initial treatment for cancer) are easily extrapolated extensions of the emergency services role of a hospital

An alternative conception suggests that the hospital is a community resource for caring. Hospitals are already the principal gathering place for professionals, technicians, equipment, and support services that can be focused on packaging an individual's care in an infinite variety of ways. And when more than one hospital in a community implements this concept, neighboring hospitals with similar programs compete for patients and resort to public and professional advertising of service amenities, such as better meals, more attractive rooms, or better staff, in order to attract patients. These efforts to market the use of a particular hospital, much as various brands of toothpaste, are promoted to the public through marketing strategies. Nevertheless, as a general concept the hospital as a community resource is a particularly appropriate one for serving older adults. The hospital, while being primarily the setting for acute care, can also play a role in the overall health care of an individual. In order to do this well, a hospital would have to recognize and respond to the complexity of adaptive needs that are typically observed in older adults, needs that are biopsychosocial in nature. With the increasing longevity of the aging populations throughout the world, we are with increasing frequency being confronted also with patients who are frail. Frailty in older adult patients taxes the skills of clinicians and policy makers alike, because it is arguable whether frailty per se is a medical condition at all. Fortunately for frail elderly persons who encounter physicians and hospitals, they usually have at least one diagnosable condition in order to justify medical ministration and often hospitalization. Otherwise their inability to function would in itself give physicians and hospitals no clear role in responding.

One can imagine melding these two concepts so that the hospital is a specialized center for acute and emergency care and is also a coordinating center for community services. This melding is easier to conceptualize than it is to organize and finance. Perhaps the critical missing component is health care leadership that is motivated and skilled enough to pursue such an outcome.

SALIENCE OF MEDICAL LEADERSHIP

Physicians must play a key role in reshaping geriatric care. They have participated in advances in public health and in the related aging of populations, which have ensured a remarkable shift from acute illness to chronic illness as the dominant health problem in developed societies. This shift in the spectrum of disease requires the emergence of new patterns of care. The emphasis on diagnosis must be amended to give greater attention to functional status, particularly when the patient is an older adult. The traditional motivation to cure must be complemented by the idea that caring rather than curing is the reality of later life, and that maximization of function is the most appropriate goal to achieve. Some find this relatively simple notion difficult to manage. While the idea is simple enough, the implications for patient care are profound. One of the implications is that physicians and hospitals can neither by themselves provide appropriate geriatric care, nor can they provide it at a politically acceptable price.

EMPHASIS ON FUNCTIONING

An approach to care that emphasizes comprehensive functioning is most appropriate for older adults. And this in turn puts unique pressure on hospitals and physicians. Although inpatient stays are often needed for diagnosis and intervention in acute illnesses and for management of acute episodes in chronic disorders, the hospitalization of the older adult is not an end in itself. In geriatric care, hospitalization provides an opportunity for determining the patient's longer-term needs and prognosis, and for setting the stage for continued care once the patient is discharged. But hospitalization is at its best only a prelude to living in the community with the maximum feasible degree of independence.

Taking a comprehensive view of the older person's functioning and potential for functioning, which is fundamental to good geriatric care, challenges the prevailing hospital culture, however. This broader view necessitates a shift in perception, from the hospital as the dominant or perhaps even the sole locus of activity in health care to the hospital as only one part of a caring community. A preference for long life and the belief in high technology as a way to achieve this outcome have led to a heavy reliance on expensive technology in support of health care. Paying for new technology and being reimbursed for its use are key parts of the management strategy of virtually every major hospital in this country. Investing in caring services has appeared to be more difficult for hospitals to endorse with enthusiasm. New opportunities for financing community-based geriatric care through Medicare have done little to generate enthusiasm for developing networks of such services as home health and home helps, day care, or respite care. Even when community-based services exist, these services are frequently uncoordinated and even chaotic. The individual older person consequently requires a case-management specialist to assist in coordinating care that is offered by multiple agencies. As a result, alternatives to hospitalization have not routinely proved to reduce total health care costs.

OPPORTUNITIES FOR RESHAPING GERIATRIC CARE

The hospital has a remarkable opportunity to participate in reshaping care of older adults. Whether the hospital is or should be the centerpiece in a system of geriatric care can be debated. But the hospital will unquestionably play a vital role. The hospital is where most elderly now turn when they are sick or functionally incapacitated. Within the hospital itself, the conflict between the curative strategy and the orchestration of total care—often referred to simplistically as high tech versus high touch—needs to be and is being carefully reviewed at many levels by senior hospital administrators, physicians, nurses, and aides. Developing a sound philosophy of geriatric care is surely an urgent task for hospital leadership as a network of complementary services is being designed and implemented. The issue is not whether hospitals have an important role in geriatric care, but rather is a specification of that role.

The establishment of special inpatient units for geriatric care within hospitals is one expression of a philosophy of care, but such units are necessarily a limited statement of what is required. A comprehensive view of human functioning should pervade a hospital, not just a special unit, and should lead logically to a consideration of how a patient's discharge from the hospital optimally leads the patient back to the community. And, because most acute interventions in a hospital are followed by a period of recovery during which future care plans for return to the community need to be made, a more comprehensive patient-oriented pattern of patient care is indicated that stresses, at best, that most patients can and will live most of their days outside a hospital.

ILLUSTRATING A PHILOSOPHY OF CARE

Excellent examples of how hospitals can adapt to the changing needs of older adults and provide community leadership for reshaping geriatric care are found in the Program of Hospital Initiatives in Long-Term Care, supported by the Robert Wood Johnson Foundation of Princeton, New Jersey. The program encourages and reinforces interest in the implementation of a sound philosophy of geriatric care. In this program, 24 hospitals planned and initiated a variety of mechanisms for helping hospitalized older patients with their discharge plan and posthospital recovery period at home. In addition, by developing a variety of relationships with other support systems (e.g., home health care, Area Agencies on Aging, homemaker services, day care, family counseling, social and community services agencies), the hospitals have demonstrated how to play a crucial role in ensuring cooperative efforts to promote and maintain the best functional status of the older adult following hospitalization. The partnerships that have emerged between hospitals and community agencies have also helped prevent or facilitate hospital readmission as is appropriate to the patient's needs. Because the hospitals have virtually all adapted a case (or service) management approach to the older adults they serve, the likelihood of effective follow-through on the discharge plan is substantially heightened. In these demonstrations, the ability of the physicians to orchestrate and manage the ongoing comprehensive care of patients also is clearly enhanced because the case manager remains in contact with the former patient for months or years.

This program to encourage innovations in comprehensive long-term care has been successful in most of the hospitals and communities in which it was undertaken. Physicians, although initially slow to accept it because so many other changes were occurring at this time, have become supportive as they perceive the improvement in patient care that has typically occurred. And they have been pleased to discover how much an effective case manager can contribute to achieving appropriately comprehensive care. Nurses and social workers have had occasional difficulty in working out their respective roles as case managers, and the hospital discharge planning groups have occasionally experienced overlap in function. But these issues also have been worked out administratively. Such issues have been resolved differently in individual hospitals. This is not surprising because experienced administrators know that in complex organizations different strategies work equally well in different circumstances when implemented by skilled leaders. The most compelling evidence of the success of the Robert Wood Johnson program is that administrators have been supportive, and a surprising number of the initial group of 24 hospitals are planning to keep the programs intact, despite lack of specific new funding or reimbursement. The value to patients in participating hospitals and the attendant good will generated in the communities, as well as a recognition of the effectively broadened role of the hospital, are appreciated by those institutional leaders who embarked upon the experiment 4 years ago.

NURSING HOMES

The importance of nursing homes in the care of functionally impaired older adults is illustrated by the number of available beds. In the United States, there are currently more beds in nursing homes than the total number of beds in acute–care hospitals. The nursing home is a distinctive but not exclusive product of the organization of health care in the United States. Nursing homes in this country are primarily in the private sector (not owned by government), are predominantly occupied by disabled older adults, and have flourished only since Medicare and Medicaid legislation in 1965. Medicare envisioned a limited role for short-term transitional care between hospital and home, but proscribed long-term care in nursing. Medicaid was another matter. Medicaid permitted long-term care in nursing homes and helped generate a large industry.

The 1983 legislation of prospective payment of hospital care based on Diagnosis Related Groups (DRGs) was enacted specifically to control the cost of hospitalization under Medicare. The legislation specifically avoided addressing nursing home and physician expenditures, but hospitals were given new reasons to limit hospital stays and to monitor the cost-generating behavior of physicians involved with older patients. One way to limit hospital-related cost is the transfer of the older patient to a less costly nursing home bed. Such a strategy is reasonable on its face, but its implementation has led to accusations that hospitals are discharging old patients "quicker and sicker" in order to save money. Although this surely occurs, no convincing systematic evidence has been presented that it happens regularly or what the consequences of early discharge for health are. Experienced observers of geriatric hospital care might consider one day less of hospitalization a good thing if the hospital involved has a poor philosophy of geriatric care. However, until reassuring evidence is in, the behavior of hospitals that have vertically integrated organizationally in order to have a nursing home of their own to which geriatric patients can be discharged is reasonably suspect.

AT THE END OF LIFE

In this century our image of the hospital has been transformed to an optimistic one of a place one goes not to die but to be cured and to live. And, in fact, nowadays many more people are discharged from hospitals alive than dead. Yet the fact remains that most individuals, particularly older ones, are likely to die in a hospital. The hospice movement, which has presented a reasonable alternative to dying in a conventional hospital, has not changed this fact.

Hospitals are very expensive places to die. An oft-quoted and reliable statistic is that the 5% of Medicare enrollees who die each year generate about a third of the annual expenditures. Clearly the therapeutic optimism that replaced therapeutic nihilism in geriatrics in recent decades is sometimes expressed as therapeutic relentlessness. The technological imperative in medical care can and does generate relentless interventions and some very large bills.

Yet the ethical dilemmas associated with judicious decisions not to begin or to terminate care for sick older adults must not be underestimated. Our society has shown little enthusiasm for ethical discussions intended to identify public consensus. We probably have no right to force responsibility for such decisions on hospitals, at least not without sending clear signals that we entrust this leadership with the right as well as with the obligation to develop publicly stated rules for deciding.

PERSONNEL DEVELOPMENT AND TRAINING

The case for specialized training for health professionals who care for older adults has been made often and effectively in the past decade in the United States and much earlier in the United Kingdom and Sweden (see Chapters 4 and 6 in this volume). Much less consensus has developed nationally and internationally regarding whether geriatrics should be a subspecialty of medicine requiring formal credentials and a recognized subspecialty within nursing, social work, clinical psychology, rehabilitation, and so on.

In the United Kingdom the decision appears to have been to

establish a specialty, the *geriatric consultant,* and to worry about the training and credentials after the fact. Canada and the United States have proceeded cautiously and have discussed a specialty in geriatrics largely in terms of demonstrated competence to care for the older patient, rather than emphasizing geriatrics as a separate subdiscipline. In nursing, a case has been made for the geriatric nurse practitioner, particularly in the nursing home (see Chapter 9). But in general, discussion of geriatrics as a specialty has been politely muted in the discussion among various health care professionals.

At least two factors contributed importantly to caution in estimating the current and future need for health professionals to serve aging populations. How many of what kinds of professionals are needed and where they should be trained are contingent on some consensus about the organizational context in which professionals will practice. Another contingency is consensus about whether the focus of geriatrics is on older adults generally or only in subsets of the very old, very frail elderly. The absence of consensus on these two points makes implementation of a national policy on geriatric manpower unlikely in the United States in the near future.

INSIGHTS FROM THE SYMPOSIUM

Presentations in the symposium illustrated particularly well the limited consensus in developed countries regarding how best to organize, to finance, and to deliver efficiently and effectively health care for older adults. In the complex network of hospital and community health and welfare services that older persons require, hospitals clearly have a role to play. What is less clear is whether hospitals should be the hub, coordinator, and controller of the required network of services. In the United Kingdom and in Sweden, physicians tend to be comfortable with the centrality and dominance of hospitals in geriatric health care. The ambivalence in the United States is illustrated well by Kane (Chapter 2) and Vladeck (Chapter 3). Vladeck is probably correct in observing that the average community hospital is de facto a geriatric institution competing to survive in a competitive market. Marketing of services is required by this kind of environment, and Stanley Brody (Chapter 8) believes such marketing is not all bad if the exercise develops perceptive organizational leaders who evaluate the effectiveness as well as the efficiency of their operations. But, Kane asks, should hospitals be in charge or simply be another player in the contest for controlling the organization of geriatric services? The answer is not obvious.

Cumulatively, the chapters of this volume establish two important facts about how we are likely to ask and then to answer questions about the distinctive role of hospitals in geriatric care. First, the organization of health care and hospitals is deeply embedded in the sociocultural history of the societies in which we observe them. Few professionals in Britain and Sweden can remember a time before a national health system of health care in which the dominant roles of hospitals and physicians were mandated by legislation that confirmed public consensus. Moreover, in these societies, the practice of geriatric medicine is in a sense the practice of good medicine. Canada has now had national health insurance long enough to confirm with confidence that geriatric medicine is an integral part of the health care system. Physicians and hospitals are expected to treat health as a social good and a social responsibility. And, although provinces have some discretion in how they organize geriatric care, such care is unquestionably to be integrated with comprehensive policies related to income and housing.

The dominant perceptions, observed in other societies, of where responsiblity for geriatric care resides puts in sharp relief the ambivalence found in the United States. In this country we tend to think of health care as an economic as well as a social good, and in recent years we have reaffirmed a preference for emphasizing the economic dimension. Our mixed feelings about where responsibility for geriatric care lies has contributed to a lack of sustained organizational leadership to propose solutions for dealing effectively as well as efficiently with geriatric care.

The symposium also illustrated particularly well that how geriatric care is organized and financed is ultimately a political question. The temptation in discussing how to achieve a particular organizational outcome is to dwell on technically adequate solutions that appeal to organizational specialists. In fact, effective solutions to organizational problems ultimately depend on achieving solutions that are politically tolerable if not appealing. It is this that bothers Anne Somers in the final chapter (Chapter 10). Although she has a preference for national health insurance, she does not seem hopeful. She will settle for the assurance that ambivalence in the United States regarding hospitals does not lead to mindless political hostility toward hospitals.

INVENTING THE FUTURE

Hospitals in the United States are changing. Economic and social imperatives concomitant with the aging of the population and requirements for more health care at controlled costs are challenging both the way health care is organized and the way health care institutions function. Clearly there is emerging an increased cadre of physicians, other health care professionals, and community social service organizations that recognize the need for a better integration of hospitals and community-based care and for better use of health and social interventions. This is an issue not only of structural change but also of conceptual change. The practice of geriatrics lies not simply in the recognition that the aging person has a somewhat altered physiology and a concomitantly different set of clinical laboratory standards, or a more complex pattern of coexisting diseases, and reacts differently to treatments. The practice of adequate medical care for older persons must involve the recognition that a different style of practice is needed. This style of practice would appreciate the range of variables that affect functional capacity and incorporate into patient management a similar range of nonmedical adaptive approaches—from prostheses to socialization, day care, homemaker services, and "friendly visitors." This reconceptualization must involve acceptance by physicians of the equivalent roles of other professionals outside of medical care and must help articulate the contributions of the various institutions required in providing the spectrum of care individuals and the caring families must have.

Finally, it should be recognized that the problems of providing hospital-based health care to the elderly are only a subset of the problems in providing health care to everyone. Comprehensive national health insurance may not be in the immediate future of the United States. But the nation is unlikely to achieve an adequate system of geriatric health care until this occurs. Future strategy not only needs to develop an alternative structure for Medicare to provide for long-term care and for community-based caring, but also needs a program for financing and restructuring health care for the entire population.

REFERENCES

Rabin, D. L., & Stockton, P. (1987). *Long-term care of the elderly: A factbook.* New York: Oxford University Press.

2

The Hospital and Geriatrics: Can a Medical Center Be Happy at the Periphery?

Robert L. Kane

Any discussion of the hospital's role in the care of the elderly must acknowledge the heterogeneity of both players. No discussion of geriatric health care can avoid mentioning the artificial nature of a term like *the elderly*. The hospital's role will vary substantially with the specific group addressed. Younger, well elderly will make different demands of and derive different benefits from the hospital than will the older, frailer elderly. For these latter individuals, the hospital represents a critical juncture on a path to either avoiding or developing disability.

This definitional distinction may be approached from several perspectives. The epidemiologist talks about populations at risk and contrasts those needing simple care with those needing complex care. The marketing director will see differentially desirable customers; the desirability depends in large measure on the nature of the payment system. In a fee-for-service system, the big spenders make the best customers. The greater the pathology, the greater the revenue generated. In a fixed-payment system, the reverse applies. The most desirable customers are those who need the least done, especially if you charge each customer the same price. Small wonder that hospitals are now looking at the elderly as the demographic area of greatest customer growth and are eagerly anticipating the chance to entice the well elderly.

Most of the elderly are very functional, but some need substantial amounts of assistance. According to the 1979 National Health Interview Survey, the number of adults per 1000 who needed assistance from another person in one or more basic physical activity or home management tasks ranged from 70 in the 65-to-74-year-old age group to 436 in the 85-and-over group (Feller, 1983). In a similar fashion, data from the National Medical Care Utilization Expenditure Study indicate that in 1980 over 60% of the elderly spent less than $500 per year on health expenditures (interestingly, this proportion did not vary with age); however, 10% of the elderly spent over $3500 per year during that same year (Kovar, 1983).

This presentation will address primarily the more disabled elderly, those presenting with the newly familiar geriatric paradigm of multiple, simultaneous, interactive problems from various domains that lead to the loss of autonomous function. Appropriate geriatric care must combine careful medical evaluation to identify and treat remediable medical problems with attention to the physical, social, and psychological environment that will minimize functioning despite disability. For such people, it is virtually impossible to imagine no role for the hospital. The question is what role.

The other major observation addresses the context of these comments. The approaches considered for the hospital reflect the culture of the society around it. The concerns raised in this paper are very American and may not apply to the experience or the philosophy of other countries. Ours is a country that celebrates its entrepreneurial spirit. It is the stuff of our heroes, but it is also the basis for our litigation. Programs developed in the U.S. must be exported with care, and conversely anyone who attempts to import health care notions from abroad must have a clear picture of the relevant social customs in the locale where such notions originate.

In the United States we have moved from a concern about needs for medical care to an obsession with cost control. The language of contemporary discussion is filled with the jargon of economics and management, not of medicine (Alper, 1984). One might list the priorities of the 1960s as ACCESS, QUALITY, and cost. In the 1980s they have become COST, quality, and access.

THE HOSPITAL AS SUN OR SATELLITE

American medicine is undergoing a Copernican revolution. The hospital's role as the center of a health care solar system is being challenged. This restructuring of the system does not deny the hospital's importance in health, but it does threaten the centrality of its role. Hospitals have already responded and will respond in varying ways to this shift.

The nature of the discussion about providing health and social services has changed dramatically since the 1960s. We have moved from a profound belief in the credo of Roemer's Law (i.e., hospital supply generates demand) to a new heresy of open competition. Hospitals are previously unshakable giants who now appear to have an unsteady financial foundation (Schwartz et al., 1985). The relative importance of access, quality, and cost has been effectively revised. The emphasis on cost control has important implications for hospitals. Obviously the change in payment to a per-case basis dramatically revises strategies and incentives for linking acute and long-term care. This linkage is reinforced by government interest in expanding the system of prospective payment to tie more closely together payments for hospital and posthospital care.

From another perspective, the definition of catastrophic care has been modified to emphasize the important role of long-term care in the overall cost picture. Here again, the argument is proffered for linking more tightly hospital and long-term management (Zook et al., 1981) because costly episodes of long-term care are assumed typically to begin in the hospital. That institution is the logical place for a system of care to assign responsibility for initiating and planning necessary care.

Although it is tempting to attribute the hospital's change of heart about long-term care to the recent imposition of Medicare's prospective payment system (PPS), a shift was already underway before that policy (Starr, 1983). The pre-PPS movement from the hospital to the medical center simply predated the post-PPS move from medical center to health corporations interested in the vertical integration of acute and long-term care services. The issue at hand is not whether a transformation in geriatric care will occur but what it will look like and who will come out on top. Although hospitals will need to change their styles if they are to grow, the hospital as hospital is very likely to remain a major force in health care. The question is whether it is willing to change its style enough to remain in control, or whether it prefers to continue to play its familiar role but to play it as a part of a larger enterprise it does not control. As we examine this issue, we might want to keep in mind an important policy question: What is best for whom? There are a number of constituencies to consider and all of them will not necessarily be best served by any one particular approach.

The hospital is inexorably linked to long-term care. Even before the era of DRGs, a patient's hospital discharge itself was a significant predictor of the imminent or eventual need for long-term care in a nursing home or at home. Conversely, persons identified as long-term care clients are likely to make greater use of hospitals than are those not so designated. For example, the calculations for average-area-per-capita costs (AAPCC) for Medicare Part A give additional weight to an individual's status as a nursing home resident, especially for those under age 85. Compared to those who are in the community and not on welfare, the ratio is 2 to 3 times the base rate (Leutz et al., 1985).

THE HOSPITAL'S TRACK RECORD IN LONG-TERM CARE

Although the elderly have been promoted as a lucrative market (Brody & Persilly, 1983), hospitals have been slow to play a very active role in long-term care (Campion, Mahoney, & Bang, 1984). Moreover, the relationship between the hospital and the long-term care system has been stressful. Much of this stress can be attributed to the differences in funding streams and styles of operation. Whereas hospitals look to Medicare, long-term care looks more heavily to Medicaid. Investments of effort that are financially supported by one payer are not likely to be enthusiastically pursued if they ultimately benefit another. The hospital's initial and more enthusiastic sponsorship of home health agencies illustrates the potential of a merged funding stream, or at least one dominated by a single payer.

Closely tied to the source of funding is the institution's style of operation. Can a hospital that is used to going first-class adjust to flying tourist? The hospital has traditionally behaved like an executive with an expense account, or like a defense contractor. In matters of life and death, only the mean count costs. Long-term care, by contrast, is viewed as a less worthwhile endeavor; the benefits are less obvious. Thus the rationale for restraining costs is more salient. When efforts are made to impose some form of cost-benefit analysis, especially when a human capital approach is used, the long-term care programs are generally disadvantaged (Avorn, 1983).

The hospital's role as an entry point into long-term care has produced inconsistent behavior. There is a general feeling that hospital discharge planners give more emphasis to moving the patient out of the hospital than to considering what situation is best for the patient. Studies of nursing home placement from hospitals suggest a wide variation in discharge criteria (Kane & Matthias, 1984). Appropriate long-term care is a complex and very dynamic process. Studies of the natural history of nursing home patients indicate an active interchange between the hospital and the nursing home, with some patients moving back and forth as many as six times in 2 years (Lewis et al., 1985).

The hospital's failure to play a more responsible role in avoiding unnecessary institutionalization is particularly regrettable because the knowledge is at hand to do better. A recent randomized trial of a specialized unit designed to achieve this very purpose, the geriatric evaluation unit, has demonstrated that substantial benefits expressed as either reduced mortality, reduced institutionalization, or increased functioning can be achieved at a cost that is offset by subsequent savings by one year of discharge (Rubenstein et al., 1984). Such care can also save hospital costs. Anderson and Steinberg (1984) estimate that 22% of Medicare hospitalizations were followed by a readmission within 60 days of discharge.

Better assessment and closer linkages with community agencies could do much to forestall such events.

The advent of the Medicare prospective payment system (PPS) has influenced the nature of the hospital's role in the care of the elderly. In some cases, trends that were already established have been accentuated. In others, new relationships have been forged. The case-based payment approach provides stronger motivation to move patients out of the hospital as quickly as possible. The pressure to discharge has never been greater (except perhaps for totally unreimbursed care). Any thoughts of comprehensive geriatric assessment are far less tenable under such auspices. But PPS has had positive effects as well. Linkages between acute and long-term care have become closer. Hospitals have begun to option nursing home beds and to operate long-term care services in order to assure access for discharges.

CHANGES IN HOSPITAL STRATEGIES

Hospitals are now confronting a very different environment with more competition and more cost-consciousness (Levey & Hesse, 1985). The jargon of the business world is heard more frequently, with allusions to market share and the bottom line. At the same time, there appears to be a growing erosion of faith in doctors (Mechanic, 1985). The physician is viewed as being less compassionate and less interested in patients as people. By association at least, the hospital will similarly lose prestige, and its traditional role as the natural leader of sociomedical care will be threatened.

Hospital responses to the new competitive pressures have varied widely. Some institutions have embarked on major expansion programs into a variety of areas; others have tried to identify especially profitable ventures and to market services to specifically targeted clientele in an effort sometimes termed *niche-picking*.

At the same time that changes have been occurring in the hospital milieu, other changes have transpired in the world around it. Various forms of prepaid care are being offered. With the new regulations legislated for HMOs under Medicare, the inducements to develop new forms of health service delivery for elderly persons will be even greater. Some of these newer configurations are already attempting to link more closely health and social services, such as the social health maintenance organizations (SHMOs). As more competition develops, social services of varying types may be used increasingly as a marketing tool, especially to attract the well elderly.

These new forms of care are as often based around other community organizations as around the hospital. The hospital is often an active participant, perhaps a catalyst in spurring the formation of the new corporate entity, but it may emerge as a contractor rather than as a managing partner.

Freedman (1985) describes the "industrialization" of health care, as corporations respond to the growth in health care costs by organizing their own systems of care. He envisions a new supplier of health services developing as business coalitions combine to negotiate mass purchases of health services: the megacorporate health care delivery system.

At the same time, a major national economic shift is occurring. America is undergoing a major economic transformation from a product economy to one based heavily on services. One hears frequent reference to such concepts as corporate diversification. Corporations have begun to enter widely various fields of human services in addition to their primary retail roles. Perhaps the most visible example is the nation's largest retailer, Sears, which now offers a wide variety of human services and has recently entered the durable medical products movement.

Two corporate forces appear to be colliding. From one direction we note the growth of health corporations that are integrated both vertically and horizontally. Using combined resources for growth and capital expansion, such firms are moving to diversify by entering other related fields, such as housing. From the other pole, more traditional corporations are now eyeing health care as an area for investment.

IS THERE SUCH A THING AS A HOSPITAL?

In considering the appropriate role of the hospital in the larger system of health care for the elderly, we need to recognize the heterogeneity of the institution. Hospitals differ greatly in size and sponsorship. Are we pursuing a single policy designed to fit all hospitals, or do we focus on some model hospital? The growth in proprietary hospitals, for example, may provoke anxieties that a policy designed for a community hospital might be turned to serve other purposes in the hands of a profit-making institution.

Similarly, hospitals may play different roles in different settings. The rural facility may be a natural source of organizational expertise, but in a densely populated urban area there may be a variety of agencies vying for the leadership role. A highly specialized, sophisticated tertiary care facility will likely assign a very different priority to developing a community service network than would a hospital that provides more general care.

Hospital parlance has been dotted with terms like *vertical integration, horizontal integration,* and *diversification.* As more and more hospitals become linked as parts of corporate structures, there is some cause to question the strength of their commitment to their primary service community. The tendancy toward centralized management, with the imposition of standardized practices and accountability to a distant corporate headquarters, must be balanced against the need to recognize the importance of responsiveness to local community needs in order to maintain market share.

Sometimes it is difficult to recognize a hospital. Diversification of mission and a search for new markets has led hospitals into a variety of new ventures. Hospitals have become health centers. An increasing proportion of their work is done on an outpatient basis. Often they may more closely resemble a motel attached to a professional office building than the familiar standard fixture recognizable as a community hospital. The contemporary hospital may offer a broad spectrum of services, including such things as wellness and health promotion, alcohol rehabilitation, treatment for eating disorders, and housing.

Some have criticized this broadened agenda as unnecessary medicalization of social problems. Some personal and social problems have now been relabeled as diseases, a transformation that may affect their social significance and their potential for coverage under health insurance. However, the critics of this medical approach are quick to note that the increased cost of the treatment is not necessarily accompanied by any greater effectiveness. Programs that used to be inexpensive as voluntary efforts using nonprofessionals have now been professionalized and actively marketed, but the success rate for treatment remains the same. Why, then, they ask, should one program charge a great deal under health insurance coverage, while another provides very similar services at much less cost but cannot recover even those costs because it is not a medical entity?

Hospitals have thus shown great flexibility in adapting to new opportunities, but the flexibility may be greater in marketing than in changing basic patterns of operation. Such experience suggests that if they become more active in long-term care (LTC), hospitals may redefine social problems as medical diseases and follow the same pattern of more expensive but no more efficacious care.

SHOULD THE HOSPITAL BE IN CHARGE?

Undoubtedly the safest answer to the question of who should control geriatric health care services is, "It depends." Campion, Bang, and May (1983) have urged hospitals to get more involved in long-term care. They base their position on seven related points: (1) Hospitals have a historic mission of supporting and caring for the elderly and chronically ill; (2) hospitals are points of access to the system; (3) the elderly are disproportionately high utilizers of hospital care; (4) hospitals can target resources to those most at risk for expensive hospitalization; (5) hospitals could induce physicians to intervene in nursing homes (and presumably in the community) to prevent unnecessary hospitalizations; (6) discharge from the hospital could be facilitated; and (7) economic survival of the hospital demands better linkage with LTC.

Such an overview is clearly hospitocentric. A more balanced view can recognize both advantages and liabilities in the hospital's playing a more active role in community care of the elderly. Table 2-1 attempts to summarize some of the major arguments for and against the centrality of the hospital in the care of the elderly, especially the chronically ill, dependent elderly who typify long-term care clients.

TABLE 2-1 Arguments for and against a Greater Role for Hospitals in Long-Term Care

For	Against
Existing administrative structure	Medical model—Failure to value social service
Motivation	Expensive
High-quality standards	Overly professional
Frequent point of contact	Excessively technological
Good community reputation—Destigmatize problems	High administrative costs
History of flexibility	Danger of selective targeting
Access to various professionals	Principal goal to increase market share
Influence on physicians	Not adept at community work
Dominant size—Won't respond unless in control	
Relative cost of hospital care	

A glance at the table reveals an interesting point. The same attributes may often be viewed as either assets or liabilities, depending on the degree of persistence and one's own perspective. Thus, for many, the hospital represents a means of improving quality, strengthening professional input, and developing a more systematic managerial focus. But others quake at the thought of a cadre of administrators interfering with what has been viewed as a humanistic process. Although one can recognize the general lack of professional input into long-term care, there is no clear evidence that care by professionals is more effective than is humane, compassionate attention from nonprofessionals. Much of LTC is acknowledged to be low-technology care in which the attitude of the caregiver may be more important than technical skills.

One area of a needed professional involvement in the care of the dependent elderly is the role of the physician. To the extent that the hospital has coercive or persuasive powers over doctors and therefore has the potential to encourage them to pay more and better attention to their elderly patients, the hospital role is important. However, this function is not unique to hospitals. Physician groups may have more direct influence. Nonmedical groups can effectively use the leverage of direct payment to induce better performance from physicians.

Hospitals have not had a very high tolerance for social services. Although various medical leaders since Richard Cabot (1909) have extolled the importance of social work, the history of the hospital suggests that such care has remained very much an adjunctive service rather than a core service. Even early efforts to use interdisciplinary teams to deliver hospital-based community care ended up devaluing the contribution of the social worker compared to the more medically oriented team members (Silver, 1974). More recently, one finds social workers marketing a skill to the hospital administration as a means of avoiding lawsuits (Nacman, 1980) or of increasing revenue (Rosenberg & Weissman, 1980).

There is a further concern, based on a distrust of altruism. Hospital care is big business. Hospitals are likely to pursue those avenues they perceive as being in their own best interest. Reducing hospital stays may not always be in the client's best interest. Targeting service toward those most at risk for hospitalization may ignore those in need of less sophisticated but equally important support. Although it is enticing to argue that social services may reduce the need for medical care (Diamond et al., 1980), evidence to support that contention is still scarce.

Funds for increased long-term care are not likely to come out of new monies. The most likely source of such funds is acute care. In Canada, for example, the numbers of acute hospital beds have been reduced as increased resources are directed to LTC programs (Kane & Kane, 1985a). Table 2-2 presents data from these Canadian provinces to illustrate the increasing investment in LTC as the growth of hospital care is slowed. The pattern persists across the different systems of LTC programs. Reduction in effort in areas of high technology could certainly produce funds redirectable to LTC. How likely is a hospital to advocate such a strategy? Hospitals do not appear to be the best sponsors of a program designed to reduce hospital use.

If hospitals are to assume a dominant role in comprehensive care for the elderly, certain changes are in order (Campion et al., 1983). Hospital personnel are not very knowledgeable about the elderly. Despite increased interest in geriatrics over the past several years, there is still only a handful of trained geriatricians, far

TABLE 2-2 Provincial Expenditures ($ in Millions) of Nursing Home and Hospital Care (in Constant Dollars)

	Hospital	Nursing home	Hospital/ nursing home
Ontario			
1973–1974	986	105*	9.4
1982–1983	1376	190*	7.2
% change/year	4	9	.44
Manitoba			
1974	159	30	5.3
1982–1983	225	55	4.1
% change/year	5	10	.48
British Columbia			
1979–1980	701	117	6.0
1982–1983	878	167	5.3
% change/year	8	14	.56

*Includes nursing homes and extended care beds in homes for the aged.

SOURCE: Kane, R. A. & Kane, R. L. (1985a).

below the minimal numbers needed (Kane et al., 1981). Hospitals have not yet exhibited a sensitivity to the social–medical needs of the elderly (Kane, Ouslander, & Abrass, 1984). Only recently has there been any effort to restructure the hospital's physical environment in order to minimize the trauma of hospitalization (Thomas & Bobrow, 1984).

ALTERNATIVES TO HOSPITAL CENTRALITY

As has already been noted, several other types of health organizations have emerged to challenge the natural claim of the hospital to a central role in the care of the elderly. Health maintenance organizations (HMOs) have grown impressively (Mayer & Mayer, 1985) and should do well with their services for the elderly, particularly those covered by Medicare. Such organizations contract with or operate hospitals, but they are based in larger administrative structures that view the hospital as only a component of the whole. The expanded model, SHMOs, offers more long-term care benefits (Leutz et al., 1985). The initial SHMO demonstration sites illustrate the potential diversity of organizational sponsorship. One site is operated by a long-term care institution that has contracted for medical and hospital care. Another is based in a community case-management organization with similar contractual bonds to medical resources. Another is a partnership between a long-term care system and an HMO. The fourth is an expanded project within a well-established HMO.

A brief look at systems of care in other countries underlines the possibilities for mixed configuration. In the United Kingdom, a strongly regionalized health care system operated by a national health service must interface with a social service system operated and funded predominantly at a local level. Although geriatric services have been established in most district hospitals, there is wide variation in both the role of the hospital vis-a-vis the local social agencies and the degree to which that leadership comes from geriatrics (Isaacs & Evers, 1984; Rai et al., 1985).

In Canada, health services are primarily a provincial responsibility. Several provinces have developed extensive long-term care programs built on a framework of universal insurance coverage. These programs are often housed in Ministries of Health, but their thrust is primarily social. Hospital services remain independent, and long-term care is essentially contracted for as case managers identify a need for it (Kane & Kane, 1985b). Although there are some examples of effective linkages between acute hospital care and long-term care, the two spheres are not tightly coordinated. Decisions to shift resources from one sector to another are made at upper levels of government.

CONCLUSIONS

It appears that there is no major reason why hospitals should be precluded from entering into long-term care. However, there is no reason to continue the myth that hospitals are essential to such activity. The appropriate course lies in first identifying what is expected from the long-term care system and in developing a mechanism to hold providers accountable for achieving reasonable goals. Certainly an important, perhaps essential, component of such a system is the effective interface between acute care and long-term care.

The hospital is no longer a sacrosanct institution. If it decides to play an active role in LTC, it will have to reorient itself to provide a new set of services with a different style of practice. The market for hospital services cannot afford to be standoffish. Because hospitals rely on the elderly as an important source of patients, they should be willing to work with LTC agencies to develop productive relationships. The hospital's participation in LTC as a source of acute inpatient services thus should not depend on the hospital's role in controlling the LTC program.

Hospitals need to change their behavior. They need to assess their basic procedures for providing care in order to determine what they do that is potentially harmful, especially to the vulnerable venerables. Some hospitals need to bring their behavior into conformity with their advertising. It is embarrassing to read advertisements for hospitals that make them sound more like resorts, but it is unethical when these promises of personalized services are violated in daily practice.

Hospitals may not be able to control physician behavior as well as was once believed, but their environment provides important incentives that nonetheless influence physician behavior. The messages offered by the work environment are likely to be more important in determining physician attitudes toward elderly patients than is much of medical education. If the institutions emphasize and reward efforts to humanize care, to minimize the psychological trauma of hospitalization disorientation, and strive to maintain patient autonomy, they will set important models for their medical staff. Moreover, such behavior is good business if they are serious about attracting a geriatric clientele.

The hospital that views LTC as a potential marketing tool may be in for a surprise. The level of investment in LTC required may well be far larger than the extent of gain in market share afforded by the extra exposure to potential clientele. In fact, a sincere commitment to LTC may lead to an effort designed to reduce hospital use. Hospitals are thus better advised to enter LTC when they are in search of diversification rather than when they are looking for a loss-leader for marketing purposes.

When one hears of a hospital that seems to be directing its attention to LTC for altruistic reasons, there is cause for concern. Such an institution is either naive or devious. However, some hospitals may indeed appropriately view an expanded role in long-term care as in their own best interest, and some of these hospitals may happen to be in geographic areas where such a role represents a benefit to the community.

REFERENCES

Alper, P. R. (1984). The new language of hospital management. *New England Journal of Medicine, 311,* 1249–1251.

Anderson, G. F., & Steinberg, E. P. (1984). Hospital readmissions in the Medicare population. *New England Journal of Medicine, 311,* 1349–1353.

Avorn, J. (1984). Benefit and cost analysis in geriatric care. *New England Journal of Medicine, 310,* 1295–1301.

Brody, S. J., & Persilly, N. (Eds). (1983). *Hospitals and the aged: The new old market.* Rockville, MD: Aspen Systems.

Cabot, R. C. (1909). *Social service and the art of healing.* New York: Moffat, Yard.

Campion, E. W., Bang, A., & May, M.I. (1983). Why acute-care hospitals must undertake long-term care. *New England Journal of Medicine, 308,* 71–75.

Campion, E. W., Mahoney, A., & Bang, A. (1984). Acute care hospitals providing elderly and long-term care services. A survey of the Massachusetts experience. *Journal of the American Geriatrics Society, 32,* 727–733.

Diamond, L. D., & Berman, L. (1980). The social HMO—A single entry prepaid long-term care system. In J. S. Callahan & S. E. Wallace (Eds.), *Reforming the long-term care system.* Lexington, MA: Lexington Books.

Feller, B. (1983, September). Americans needing help to function at home (Advanced data from *Vital and Health Statistics* No. 92, National Center for Health Statistics, DHHS publication No. PHS 83-1250). Hyattsville, MD: U.S. Public Health Service.

Freedman, S. (1985). Megacorporate health care. *New England Journal of Medicine, 312,* 579–582.

Isaacs, B., & Evans, H. (1984). *Innovations in the care of the elderly.* Dover, NH: Croom-Helm.

Kane, R. A., & Kane, R. L. (1985a). The feasibility of universal long-term care benefits: Ideas from Canada. *New England Journal of Medicine, 312,* 1357–1364.

Kane, R. L., & Kane, R. A. (1985b). *A will and a way: What Americans can learn about long-term care from Canada*. New York: Columbia University Press.

Kane, R. L., & Matthias, R. (1984). From hospital to nursing home: The long-term care connection. *Gerontologist, 24,* 604–609.

Kane, R. L., Ouslander, J. C., & Abrass, I. B. (1984). *Essentials of clinical geriatrics*. New York: McGraw Hill.

Kane, R. L., Solomon, D. H., Beck, J. C., Keeler, E., & Kane, R. A. (1981). *Geriatrics in the United States: Manpower projections and training considerations*. Lexington, MA: Heath.

Kovar, M. G. (1983, November). Expenditures for the medical care of elderly people living in the community throughout 1980. *National medical care utilization and expenditure survey: Data report No. 4* (DHHS publication No. PHS 84-20000, National Center for Health Statistics, Public Health Service). Washington, DC: U.S. Government Printing Office.

Leutz, W. N., Greenberg, J. N., Abrahams, R., Prottas, J., Diamond, L. M., & Gruenberg, L. (1985). *Changing health care for an aging society: Planning for the social/HMO*. Lexington, MA: Lexington Books.

Levey, S., & Hesse, D. D. (1985). Bottom-line health care? *New England Journal of Medicine, 312,* 644–646.

Lewis, M. A., Cretin, S. & Kane, R. L. (1985). The natural history of nursing home patients. *Gerontologist 25*(4), 382–388.

Mayer T. R., & Mayer, G. G. (1985). HMOs: Origin and development. *New England Journal of Medicine, 312,* 590–594.

Mechanic, D. (1985). Public perceptions of medicine. *New England Journal of Medicine, 312,* 181–183.

Nacman, M. (1980). Social worker can eliminate potential risks. *Hospitals, 54*(12), 189–192.

Rai, G. S., Murphy, P., & Pluck, R. A. (1985). Who should provide hospital care of elderly people? *Lancet, I,* 683–684.

Rosenberg, G., & Weissman, A. (1981). Marketing social work services in health care settings. *Health and Social Work, 6,* 4–12.

Rubenstein, L. Z., Josephson, K. R., Wieland, G. D., English, P. A., Sayre, J. A., & Kane, R. L. (1984). Effectiveness of a geriatric evaluation unit: A randomized clinical trial. *New England Journal of Medicine, 311,* 1664–1670.

Schwartz, W. B., Newhouse, J. A., & Williams, A. P. (1985). Is the teaching hospital an endangered species? *New England Journal of Medicine, 313,* 157–162.

Silver, G. A. (1984). *Family medical care* (2nd ed.). Cambridge, MA: Ballinger.

Starr, P. (1983). *Social transformation of American medicine*. New York: Basic Books.

Thomas, J., & Bobrow, M. (1984). Targeting the elderly in facility design. *Hospitals, 58*(4), 83–88.

Zook, C. J., Moore, F. D., & Zeckhauser, R. J. (1981, winter). "Catastrophic" health insurance—A misguided prescription? *Public Interest, 62,* 66–81.

3

Hospitals, the Elderly, and Comprehensive Care

Bruce C. Vladeck

American hospitals are experiencing a period of extraordinary change. After two decades of accelerating cost inflation, the inevitable and long-awaited reaction of major payers has all but eliminated cost-based reimbursement, has begun to substantially affect utilization patterns, and has introduced new competitive forces into many hospital markets. The continuing outflow of the physician-training pipeline has created at least the potential for enormous changes in the relationships between hospitals and their medical staffs. And the technological explosion in medicine and related disciplines continues in its inherently unpredictable but invariably consequential progress.

At the same time, the continued growth—and perhaps more importantly, perception of growth—of nonprofit and, especially, for-profit hospital chains, combined with developments in capital markets and proposed changes in the tax code, have raised profound questions about the ownership and governance of health care institutions. Amid all this turbulence, it is hardly surprising that public attitudes about hospitals and hospital care, at least as reflected in actual behavior, are also increasingly confused and volatile.

Hospital managers and trustees are at least as confused and apprehensive about these developments as anyone else. They are certainly often at a loss as to how to plan for an increasingly uncertain future, and they are increasingly at risk of making ill-considered, short-sighted, even panicky decisions. Certainly, those who market the quick fix or the all-in-one panacea after a sales pitch of gloom and doom are thriving as never before.

One of the things often inadequately understood about the current environment, and inadequately considered as the basis for future planning at both the institutional and community levels, is the absolute centrality of services to the elderly in the current hospital environment, both in planning for the future and in the development of sound public policy to get us from here to there. Conversely, the developing experience in building comprehensive care systems for the elderly provides continual reminders of the central importance of appropriate and well-managed hospital care for any such system.

These assertions—that the elderly are central to the hospital system and that hospitals are central to comprehensive care—form the twin themes of this chapter. Those themes will be explored first from the perspective of the hospital, then from the perspective of the client (patient), and then from the perspective of those concerned with financing the system. These perspectives will then be brought together with some observations and recommendations for hospitals, for clients, and for public policy.

THE ELDERLY AND THE HOSPITAL

The insured, employed nonelderly population is disappearing from the hospital, or at least from its inpatient units. The extraordinary recent decline in inpatient utilization among the nonelderly—down 7.5% in admissions and 11% in total days from 1981 to 1984—is as yet largely unexplored in any rigorous way, but a lot of forces are obviously at work, all pushing in the same direction, and all likely to continue to push that way (Vladeck, 1985).

Formal utilization controls, such as preadmission certification, mandatory second surgical opinions, and incentives for outpatient surgery, imposed by employers and insurers have, no doubt, had some effect. So has the further growth in HMO enrollment, given the capacity of at least some HMOs to lower inpatient use. Perhaps more important is the growing preference of physicians, who are motivated by a concern for maintaining their incomes in markets where a relatively stable supply of patients is spread over an increasing number of physicians, to capture overhead revenues from a widening range of diagnostic and therapeutic services by having them conducted in their offices or in freestanding centers rather than in hospitals. New technologies, from digital angiography to laser surgery, help reinforce that trend.

The growing number of nonelderly people without health insurance at all who forgo or postpone hospitalization as a result must also contribute to the decline in utilization. One's suspicions must immediately be aroused by the chronological conjunction of the first major downturn in hospital utilization with a reported 50% increase in the number of uninsured persons, in a time immediately subsequent to the worst recession in 50 years. Given the continuing depression in many parts of the manufacturing sector and in many communities dependent on that sector, as well as other changes in the labor market, the trend toward increasing numbers of the uninsured is unlikely to be quickly reversed. Nor, given the behavior of hospitals in recent years and the increasing fiscal pressures they perceive themselves to be experiencing, is the relationship between lack of insurance and low utilization soon likely to alter.

Finally, it must be acknowledged that, so far as anyone can tell, the nonelderly population is getting healthier as the result of better medical care, better living standards, changes in health-affecting behaviors, and the multigenerational effects of better nutrition, vaccination, and the like. The link between health status and the use of health services remains somewhat tenuous, but there is some relationship—indeed, as Mark Blumberg has noted, perhaps more of a relationship than we have in recent years been prepared to acknowledge (Blumberg, 1984).

For years, health care analysts have pointed to utilization rates on the order of 380 days per thousand enrollees in Kaiser-

Permanente's Northern California and Oregon regions as desirable but far-fetched targets toward which other groups (in a nonelderly population averaging 800 to 1000 days per 1000 enrollees) might someday aspire. But to many (including some in Kaiser) it no longer seems obvious that Kaiser's level is an unobtainable objective for others, nor that substantially lower rates might be obtainable in well-managed systems.

At some point, of course, still further reductions in hospital use are not cost-effective, if some level of service quality is to be maintained. And many of the pressures operating to reduce inpatient utilization among the nonelderly affect the elderly as well. But in the current fad for reduced use of inpatient services, neither narrow economics nor simple logic always govern, and clearly we still have an awfully long way to fall.

The point, of course, is that the largest group of hospital users, and the only group of high users that is going to grow for the balance of this century, is the elderly. Persons 65 and over already account for roughly 40% of all inpatient days in general hospitals, and that proportion can only grow as the proportion of elderly in the population increases, as the elderly themselves age, and as utilization falls faster in younger populations. Thus the elderly are central to hospitals because they are the customers who consume the greatest single share—soon, in most hospitals, over a half—of their principal product. Moreover, the elderly comprise the only real growth market in demand for hospital services; and, as demand for hospital services continues to fall in many other parts of the population, the elderly will more and more constitute the only available new customers.

Of course, not all hospitals fully realize this yet. One watches with some bemusement the increasingly frantic scramble by hospitals in many communities to lock up market share among employed groups that do not use much inpatient care to begin with and who are committed to reducing the amount they do use, while ignoring or even taking steps that offend elderly customers. From the viewpoint of institutional strategy, this approach is analogous to that of a turn-of-the-century entrepreneur trying to corner the market on horse feed or gas lamps.

The centrality of elderly patients to hospitals is reinforced by the decision to reform Medicare reimbursement through the use of DRGs. Even in those hospitals with relatively small proportions of Medicare patients, the switch to diagnosis-based payment requires changes in medical records practices and in medical staff behaviors. In order to prosper under a DRG-based system, hospitals also need to strengthen relationships between administration and medical staff, develop new cost-accounting procedures, and strengthen quality assurance, infection control, and discharge planning activities. None of these changes are easily confined to Medicare patients, and their pervasiveness is, of course, only reinforced when other payers also adopt DRG-based payment practices, as they increasingly have.

America's community hospitals are thus de facto geriatric institutions and will become more so, whether they know it or not. The extent to which they do not know it is, indeed, reflected in some of their reported responses to the Medicare DRG system. If the anecdotal evidence that hospitals are inappropriately discharging some Medicare patients "quicker and sicker," shunning admissions of others believed to have "unprofitable" diagnoses, and underserving still others reflects patterns of actual behaviors, then those hospitals are revealing not only a fundamental misunderstanding of the economics of DRGs, but also a misunderstanding of where their future necessarily lies. Under a system of case-based payment, the principal determinant of financial outcomes for institutions operating at less than capacity must always be the number of cases they treat, and increasingly sophisticated Medicare recipients are the only plausible source of new inpatient cases.

Of course, to speak of hospitals as unitary, monolithic entities is to overlook the extent to which their behavior is really controlled by the actions of relatively autonomous professionals, especially physicians. The conception of hospitals as essentially doctors' workshops is probably less accurate now than it has been for many years, but what doctors do and how they perceive things is clearly still an important component of hospital behavior. Here, too, the elderly are increasingly central.

While geriatrics as an independent specialty remains in its early infancy in this country, care of geriatric patients comprises an ever-increasing share of what it is that most physicians *do*. If one excludes pediatricians and obstetricians, close to a third of all physician visits are made by persons 65 and older. The proportion is still higher in specialties like urology, ophthalmology, rheumatology, and so forth (Robert Wood Johnson Foundation, 1981). Similarly, because 2 in 5 hospital days involve the elderly, it means that a roughly equivalent proportion of hospital-based physician services involves geriatric patients. And physicians are facing the same demographic and socioeconomic trends as are hospitals. In other words, recognition that they are in the business of geriatric care is not something hospitals will face in contradistinction to their physicians; rather, they will need to face it jointly (and, one hopes, cooperatively).

HOSPITALS AND THE ELDERLY

If hospitals are geriatric institutions to a far greater extent than most of them have recognized, it needs to be immediately acknowledged that most of them are not very good—or, at least, have traditionally not been very good—at serving geriatric clients. The iatrogenic effects on the elderly of many standard hospital practices have been well documented (Steel, Gertman, Crescenzi, & Anderson, 1981). Ageism is still highly prevalent among the professionals and quasi-professionals who work in hospitals. And to the extent that clinical services in hospitals are still largely dominated by the implicit model of the physicians' workshop—and they still are in most places—then the continued indifference, inadequacy, or incompetence of many practicing physicians toward a range of geriatric problems is only magnified and reinforced in the inpatient setting.

The sad state of discharge planning in many hospitals is an excellent illustration of this last phenomenon. Given that the vast proportion of hospitalized elderly patients suffer from one or more chronic conditions, effective postdischarge services involve far more than arranging for nursing home placements for the small proportion of elderly patients actually requiring nursing home care. But physicians have generally been indifferent—if not downright hostile—toward formal discharge planning services and, as a result, such services have rarely received adequate attention in hospital budgetary or management decision processes. The post-DRG rediscovery of discharge planning by hospital administrators, emanating in considerable part from the misplaced obsession with length of stay, has been dangerously episodic and placement-oriented in its emphasis and even then has frequently been frustrated by the reluctance of physicians to pay much attention to it.

Nor does the establishment of specialty inpatient geriatric or geriatric evaluation units really reflect an appropriate understanding of geriatric services by hospital managers. Although such units may be extremely successful and worthwhile in themselves, they can also reinforce the misperception that the problems of geriatric patients are those of a peculiar minority. Concentrating special resources on a 20- or 30-bed unit when geriatric patients occupy 100 or 200 beds on the average day may make it harder, not easier, to service adequately those patients not on the special unit.

But even if hospitals have not in general distinguished themselves in their services to the elderly, the elderly are still stuck with the hospitals. They simply experience too much morbidity to avoid them. And, of course, the more problems an elderly person has, the more likely it is that prevailing technologies and clinical norms require that those problems be addressed through inpatient services. Almost one in five elderly persons is hospitalized at least once in any given year, and the rate of hospitalization increases, of course, pretty much monotonically with age (Aday, Fleming, & Anderson, 1984).

ISSUES AND OPTIONS

At the practical level, at least for the time being, we appear to be prepared as a matter of policy to pay from public funds for a lot of specific goods and services only to the extent they are provided to hospital inpatients. For Medicare patients, inpatient drugs and supplies are covered in full, but outpatient drugs are not covered at all. The same is true for much of social services, nonrehabilitative nursing, nutrition counseling, and so on. Indeed, payers for health care, including Medicare, will increasingly seek to make payment on the basis of broader "bundles," or packages of services. Regardless of whether that process always extends to all-inclusive bundles such as those contemplated in some especially ambitious capitation schemes, hospitals are especially well situated to adapt to this trend. In the first place, they are already accustomed to recordkeeping and billing on a per diem or per admission basis that subsumes many specific services in one global amount; social services, discharge planning, nursing, and medical records are already standard parts of hospitals' routine costs. Second, in any system of global pricing or payment, the cost of hospitalization invariably constitutes the biggest single chunk. The hospital's costs (or prices), and thus the hospital itself, unavoidably occupy a central strategic position.

The relationship of hospital prices to more inclusive pricing bundles points up an even more fundamental issue from the hospital's perspective. As we increasingly move, in one form or another, to relatively more comprehensive systems of care, the centrality of the hospital in both economic and clinical terms means that the inpatient hospital component must receive particularly focused attention. In other words, the inpatient hospital component must be effectively *managed*. For the hospitals, the strategic question is whether they will be managers or co-managers of the system, or the objects of someone else's management. They will either manage or be managed.

Perhaps most importantly, the increasing body of experience with home- and community-based long-term care services continually reminds us of the capacity of hospitals to mess up even the best-managed long-term care cases. Sooner or later, frail elderly long-term care clients are going to end up in the hospital for treatment of acute problems, and in such instances even care that is minimally adequate by prevailing professional standards may undo months of successful service in terms of functional dependency, self-esteem and self-image, management of depression, or even cognitive orientation and functioning.

Improvement in the capacity of hospitals to effectively care for elderly patients, and the realization in practice of that capacity, is thus an essential linchpin in any strategy aimed at improving health and medical services to the elderly, whether or not the hospital is perceived or sought after as the hub of the service system. One can begin from the position that, because of their track record and the institutional pressures that work against optional geriatric services, hospitals should not serve as the foci of comprehensive long-term care or community geriatric systems. However, one cannot construct or maintain such systems without adequately incorporating improved hospital services.

And in many communities, even given poor hospital track records, there may be compelling reasons to encourage the choice of the general hospital as the hub of the community care system. For the long-term care population, hospitals are by far the predominant entry points for nursing home and formal home care. That is not just an artifact of reimbursement or bureaucratic practices; for the marginal, at-risk frail elderly, need for formal long-term care services is frequently triggered by a particular event or crisis of the sort that often requires a hospital stay.

For all geriatric services, general hospitals, notwithstanding their very consequential limitations, do constitute in many communities the most significant aggregations (and aggregators) of professional talents and skills. Hospitals are where most of the nurses, therapists, and health-oriented social workers are employed, and where most of the doctors congregate. Physicians actually prefer providing services at the hospital to providing service in community care settings, nursing homes, or their patients' homes. Inadequate though they may be, hospitals also possess a range of managerial and financial resources (or at least processes) far exceeding those available to most other health care providers.

Now that the misunderstanding of DRG economics has made vertical integration of services such a fad in hospital management, hospitals will increasingly seek to become providers of at least a broader spectrum of geriatric services, regardless of whether their doing so makes qualitative or organizational sense. Rather than resisting this trend, advocates of better services for the elderly might do better by seeking to capitalize on it as a vehicle for beginning the massive but essential task of educating hospital managers, physicians, nurses, and other professionals in how to do a better job of caring for older adults.

FINANCING

The crude economics of the continued graying of America, especially of the aging of the 65-and-older population, so frightens many policymakers that they try not to think about the policy issues at all. We are now spending something on the order of $5000 to $6000 per capita, on average, for health services for the elderly, and per capita expenditures continue to increase almost monotonically with age after 55 or 60. If the demographic projections are right and with current investments we are still not adequately serving the needs of many of the elderly with the most intractable chronic problems such as Alzheimer's disease, then as a society we risk running out of money with which to pay for services—unless payment reforms such as DRGs prove over time to be much more effective than anyone now really expects.

CENTRAL ROLES OF HOSPITALS

The only escape from the inevitable playing out of these growth curves and related costs for services is through the hospital, in at least three respects. First, better in-hospital care should reduce morbidity, as well as treat the morbidity that remains more effectively. Second, better community and medical care can significantly reduce the use of inpatient care, thus generating a potential economic dividend that can be redirected to other services or to serving a growing population. Third, if we plan and manage effectively, excess hospital capacity in human resources and physical plant can be redeployed to nonacute services rather than be abandoned, thus permitting the expansion of such services at marginal rather than incremental average cost.

Taking these points in turn, the treatment of acute illnesses in elderly hospital patients—which, it must be emphasized, is usually quite successful—too often generates other illnesses or disabilities. To the extent that such complications must be treated in the course of the same hospitalization, as in the case of postoperative or nosocomial infections, then the incentives in the DRG system permit the immediate capture of savings from better care by the institution itself. Over time those savings should become available at the systemic level as well. But if 2 or 3 days of additional acute confinement were used to provide effective occupational therapy, caregiver training, or social service planning, the risk of rehospitalization might be reduced. If this is in fact the case, our current incentives for early discharge under the DRG strategy may be quite perverse and need to be altered. Some variant of capitation-based financing may be a preferred alternative (Lohr, Brook, Goldberg, Chassen, & Glennan, 1985).

The bigger source of savings lies in reducing utilization of hospitals for acute care at existing levels of morbidity or disability. For elderly populations, the best way to do that probably involves a mixture of HMO-like utilization controls and effective case management, as well as community-based care for the chronically ill. Proponents of social/HMOs, for example, project potential reductions in acute hospitalization of as much as 25% (Leutz et al., 1985). Evaluating those savings at marginal cost suggests a potential savings of $5 billion to $6 billion in 1985. Those dollars could buy a lot of home care, rehabilitation, or outpatient drugs.

At the moment, the principal barriers to seeking such savings from reduced inpatient care lies in the web of intergovernmental fiscal relations. States are reluctant to spend new dollars on community services or on case management in order to save Medicare federal inpatient dollars; Medicare is reluctant to expand home care services that might reduce the need for state-financed nursing home services. Fragmentation of funding frustrates integration of services so that, paradoxically, the desire of each payer to minimize its own expenditures prevents reduction in total costs. This problem is not so much operational or conceptual as it is political, and adequate political will to resolve it is lacking. Eventually, however, this problem will have to be resolved, because the capture of savings from the acute inpatient sector will come to be recognized as a critical source of necessary funds.

Finally, as the experience with the Medicare swing-bed program demonstrates, service expansion through the redeployment of excess capacity in the acute hospital sector can be an extremely economical way of financing such expansion (Shaughnessy et al.,

1980). For this redeployment to be qualitatively satisfactory, however, hospitals and their staffs must be appropriately motivated, educated, supervised, and policed. Again, the substantive problems are primarily managerial and political, not economic.

For at least a decade, the notion of converting excess, underutilized acute hospital capacity to other services—notably long-term care—has had wide currency in the hospital field. Indeed, at one time there even existed statutory authority for the federal government to make grants and loans to encourage such conversion, although no money was ever appropriated. But the process of permanent conversion is probably far more complex and difficult than has been generally recognized.

To begin with, the reform of Medicare payment methods for acute care has not been accompanied by a concomitant change in methods of payment for long-term care services, and indeed the maintenance of older Medicare principles relative to cost allocation, cost-based pricing, and the like for nonacute services coexists awkwardly with prospective payment under DRGs (Vladeck, 1986). Under current practices, hospitals are all but forced to lose money if they convert acute capacity to long-term care for Medicare beneficiaries.

At the same time, the process of physical conversion itself is often difficult. Effective long-term care services require more space in patient areas (for common rooms, dining facilities, therapies, and so forth) while requiring, of course, less ancillary support in nonnursing areas. Physical plant standards for life safety and other construction requirements are significantly tougher for nursing homes than for hospitals. And while the reuse of existing facilities may intuitively seem cheaper, it is sometimes more economical to build from scratch.

PROVIDING SHORT-TERM LONG-TERM CARE

Most importantly, effective conversion of hospital capacity to long-term care requires a set of programmatic choices that hospitals have not, historically, been knowledgeable enough to make. In the spectrum of long-term care services available within any particular community, nursing home beds that serve essentially the same clients as do existing nursing homes are generally not the greatest need, nor are hospitals generally able to compete with free-standing nursing homes in the economical provision of largely residential or custodial services. On the other hand, many hospitals are at least potentially well equipped to meet the needs of the "short-term long-term care" population—those patients requiring, or likely to benefit from, postacute recuperative, restorative, and rehabilitative services of 15 to 60 days duration.

The growing need for such short-term long-term care (STLTC) services is increasingly being recognized not only as a critical link in the long-term care system, but one that makes particular sense for hospitals to fill (Vladeck, 1980). It must be emphasized, however, that short-term long-term care is different, on a number of important dimensions, from either acute or conventional long-term care. To do it effectively requires special admissions protocols, specially trained staff, strong nursing leadership, and special relations with medical staff. It is not something hospitals can just fall into. They must be prepared to jump—with eyes open.

In short, a qualitatively better and more comprehensive system of geriatric care in which hospitals did less but better acute care and more preacute and postacute care might well be significantly cheaper, on a per capita basis, than what we now have. If it were, we could then afford to care for ever-growing numbers without an extraordinary reallocation of total social resources.

CONCLUSIONS

To summarize, hospitals and the elderly are stuck with one another, and will increasingly be more so. As one facetious metaphor has it, when one has only lemons on hand, the wisest course is to make lemonade.

If we can get past the perceptual and emotional barriers that prevent us from recognizing that hospitals and the elderly are inevitably in the lemonade business together, then we can begin to approach more systematically and rationally the real tasks that lie before us. For we do not know nearly enough about how high-quality hospital services for elderly patients should be organized, staffed, or managed. We do not know enough about how to train an adequate supply of physicians, nurses, and others equipped to render high-quality geriatric care in the inpatient setting. It is not clear that we know what good inpatient geriatric services look like, let alone how to produce them. But if hospitals do not provide better services to geriatric patients in the future, they will then inevitably provide more inadequate services. We need to get to work.

REFERENCES

Aday, L. A., Fleming, G. U., & Anderson, R. (1984). *Access to medical care in the U.S.: Who has it, who doesn't.* Chicago: Pluribus Press.

Blumberg, M. S. (1984). At risk for hospitalization: Differences by health insurance coverage and income. In R. M. Scheffler & L. F. Rossiter (Eds.), *Advances in health economics and health services research: A research annual* (Vol. 5). Greenwich, CT: JAI Press.

Leutz, W. N., Greenberg, J. N., Abrahams, R., Prottas, J. M., Diamond, L. M., & Greenberg, L. (1985). *Changing health care for an aging society: Planning for the social health maintenance organization.* Lexington, MA: Lexington Books.

Lohr, K. N., Brook, R. H., Goldberg, G. A., Chassen, M. R., & Glennan, T. K. (1985, March). *Impact of Medicare prospective payment on the quality of medical care: A research agenda.* Santa Monica, CA: The Rand Corporation.

Robert Wood Johnson Foundation. (1981). *Special report: Medical practice in the United States.* Princeton, NJ: Author.

Shaughnessy, P. W., et al. (1980). An evaluation of swing bed experiments to provide long-term care in rural hospitals (Vol. 2). Denver: University of Colorado Center for Health Services Research.

Steel, K., Gertman, P. M., Crescenzi, C., & Anderson, J. (1981). Iatrogenic illness on general medical service at a university hospital. *New England Journal of Medicine, 304,* 638–642.

Vladeck, B. C. (1980). *Unloving care: The nursing home tragedy.* New York: Basic Books.

Vladeck, B. C. (1985). *President's letter: The poor use more: Hospitals and communities in New York City.* New York: United Hospital Fund.

Vladeck, B. C. (1986). Diagnosis related group-based hospital payment: The real issues. *Bulletin of the New York Academy of Medicine, 62,* 46–54.

4

The Distinctive Role of the Hospital in the Care of the Elderly in the United Kingdom

James Williamson

This chapter has been produced after more than a quarter century of work as a consultant in geriatric medicine and a decade as a professor of geriatrics. During this time I have on three occasions initiated and developed a comprehensive geriatric service for a defined population and, at the time of writing, I remain in active geriatric practice with responsibility for a service to approximately 20,000 persons aged 65 years and beyond.

It is to be hoped that some of the ideas and practices I have seen and adopted over this period could be applied elsewhere with success. If other persons are helped to avoid our mistakes and to emulate our successes, then this exercise will be worthwhile. It is, however, readily accepted that methods of providing geriatric care that are successful in one health care system may be inapplicable within a different system. Nevertheless, I believe that certain essential elements or principles may be formulated, and it is then up to those responsible for a health care system to adopt, adapt, and apply these principles in the most appropriate fashion. It could be argued that, if an existing system of health care cannot adopt sound principles, then it is not the principles that need to be changed but rather the system!

Does the hospital have a *distinctive* role in geriatric care and, if so, what is that distinctive role? This formulation of questions currently being asked accurately reflects the rather unsatisfactory nature of the debate about geriatric care, insofar as it tends to present the solution as being either institutional or noninstitutional. The truth, of course, is that care of the elderly is such a complex and infinitely varied affair that a whole range of services must be provided, including community services and a variety of institutions providing different levels of care matched to the needs of patients and carers.

It may be that much of the confusion and disagreement that persists in this field is due to a fundamental lack of understanding of the complexity of health care needs in old age. Very often the medical profession has tended to recognize only traditional medical problems and has failed to address other equally important aspects. This failure, as will be shown, can only provide at best a limited success—often at exorbitant cost.

SPECTRUM OF NEED/CONTINUUM OF CARE

I have previously explained the usefulness of considering the needs of the elderly as a spectrum that requires to be matched by a continuum of resources from which items may be selected to match needs as identified on the spectrum (Williamson, 1981a). For the healthy old person living in the "normal" social setting of a family, the needs are similar to those for other age groups—adequate income, housing, satisfying roles, and both family and nonfamily interaction. Moving along this spectrum we come upon the healthy old person who is beginning to experience social loss, for example, the widow with diminished family roles, frequently reduction in income, and sometimes living in an unsuitable house. Her problem will often be dealt with adequately by family action, but sometimes social services may be required. Should she develop anxiety, she may present somatic symptoms to a physician; hence good primary health care support for older adults is necessary from family doctors who are adequately trained in gerontology and in the medicine of old age. Still further along the spectrum we encounter patients with more complex needs and with multiple medical and social needs. At the far end is the heavily dependent aged person who requires constant nursing and frequent medical support.

The first requirement of adequate geriatric care, therefore, is a means of identifying need. This may be done competently by a well-trained family physician for patients at the "light" end of the spectrum; however, the matter becomes much more complex, difficult, and time consuming in situations where patients are further along the spectrum. This is one reason for having a specialized geriatric service that provides facilities for multidisciplinary team assessment by persons who are skilled, experienced, and highly motivated to work in such a fashion.

The second requirement of adequate geriatric care is for a balanced range of services that are speedily available and that will accurately match the identified needs. Unfortunately, most countries have to a greater or lesser degree failed to provide such a continuum. Indeed, they have often instead offered a discontinuum, in which some services are missing, some are in short supply, and some may be in excess. In addition, the provision of geriatric services often is made even more discontinuous because of gaps and barriers between services that prevent or delay the smooth transition of the patient from one aspect of care to another. These barriers may be bureaucratic. For example, the health care of an old person in the United Kingdom is the responsibility of the National Health Service, whereas the home help service is provided by local authorities financed in a different way. Other barriers may exist because of professional attitudes and prejudices, such as tensions and rivalries between doctors and nurses on one hand and social workers on the other.

The specialist geriatric service has at least crucial roles in the development and implementation of adequate care. These roles include:

1. Campaigning to achieve the elements of a balanced continuum through the identification of deficiencies and overprovision;
2. Securing effective team work, thus closing gaps, preventing overlap of services and leveling barriers; and
3. Serving as a catalyst to ensure optimum coordination of services.

These three requirements are fundamental. None of them will "just happen" unless some organization is provided to ensure their achievement. An efficient comprehensive geriatric service performs these facilitating roles without which success cannot ever be achieved. While the United Kingdom system of geriatric care may be criticized on many counts, it has been a responsible advocate for adequate geriatric services.

The geriatric services in the United Kingdom thus should be seen as being an essential part of the continuum of care but also as having a special role in ensuring the most effective use of other elements within the continuum. Hence geriatric care is not a single element but relates to various points on the continuum by acting in a catalytic fashion for all the other sources of care.

From this preamble, it is evident that an efficient geriatric service, although hospital based, must fulfill functions much wider than most hospital specialties—by providing important links with the community, by coordinating major contributions to other specialties (e.g., general practice, internal medicine, orthopedics, and psychiatry), and by placing a strong emphasis upon multidisciplinary teamwork.

DEMOGRAPHIC CONSIDERATIONS

The aging of populations in developed industrial societies is well advanced, and in many European countries the over-65s now constitute 14% to 16% of the total population. Perhaps even more alarming is the rapid aging of the population within the developing areas of the world (Myers, 1985), for which no solution seems apparent at present.

Figure 4-1 shows the picture in the United Kingdom for those aged 65+, along with projections into the next century. It will be seen that the steep increase that has taken place this century is now over and that there will be quite modest increases until 2021.

Figure 4-2 shows the projections for the 75+ group in the United Kingdom indicating that this group will continue to increase sharply until the end of the century, after which there will be a leveling off.

Figure 4-3 is the most significant of the projections, because it shows the large and continuous increase in numbers of persons aged 85+ in the United Kingdom right up to the year 2021. There is a marked preponderance of females.

It is correct to emphasize that age alone is not a good predictor of need; nevertheless, this steep and continuing increase in the most aged group has profound significance for health and social services because of the known association between age and increased risk of disability and dependence.

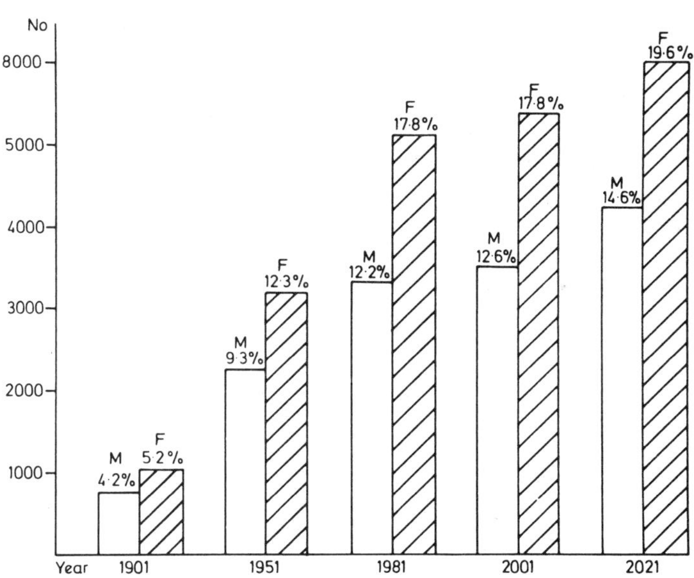

FIGURE 4-1 U.K. males and females age 65 and over (thousands) for census 1981 (percentages are of total population).

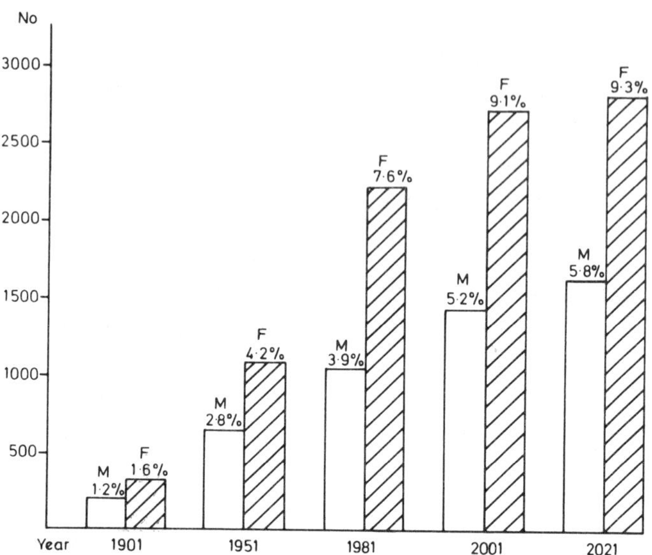

FIGURE 4-2 U.K. males and females age 75 and over (thousands) for census 1981 (percentages are of total population).

THE NATURE OF NEED IN OLD AGE

The failure to provide a continuum of resources, which has been noted, has been a fundamental problem for geriatric care in many countries. Linked with this failure is a common lack of understanding of the nature of need in old age, especially an overemphasis upon disease, often to the exclusion or neglect of other equally important factors. The following simple diagrams may help to explain this problem.

Figure 4-4 shows the traditional representation of function in relation to age. It will be seen that *growth* early in life results in very rapid increase in function; *maturity* is associated with a fairly brief maintenance of function and is succeeded by *senescence* with rapid decline. With increasing age, Figure 4-4 suggests there is increasing variability among individuals. This is, of course, an oversimplification.

Figure 4-5 illustrates the differential effect of age upon two functions. Function A (e.g., vision) is maintained for a relatively

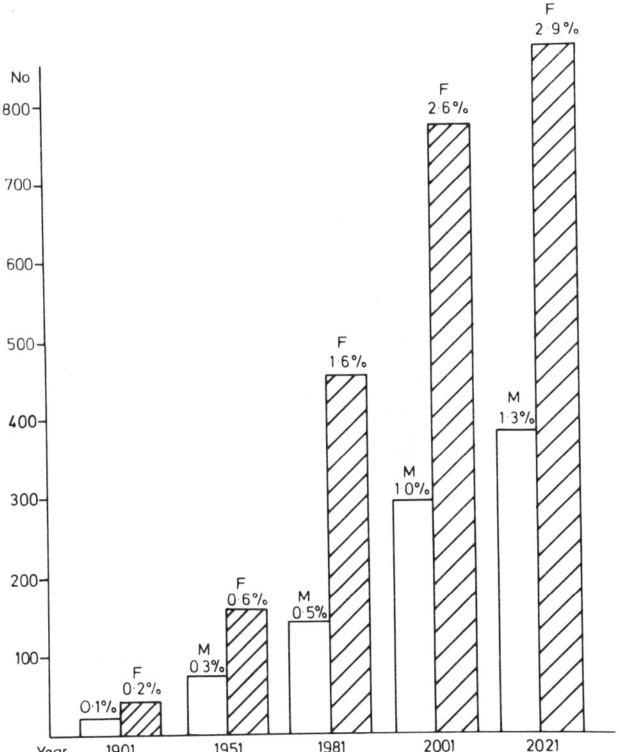

FIGURE 4-3 U.K. males and females age 85 and over (thousands) for census 1981 (percentages are of total population).

short time and thereafter declines in a linear fashion. Function B (e.g., muscle strength), on the other hand, is maintained longer before an age-related decline starts. The picture is complicated further because behavioral and environmental factors may have profound effects, as indicated in Figure 4-6.

Figure 4-6 suggests that if unhealthy behavior is adopted, the decline of a function will be steeper. The commencement of cigarette smoking, for instance, will lead to reduction in respiratory and cardiac function. Conversely, the adoption of a healthy lifestyle may improve function. Interestingly, this benefit may occur even in old age, as shown by research in Gothenburg, Sweden, which demonstrated that 70-year-old males randomly assigned to

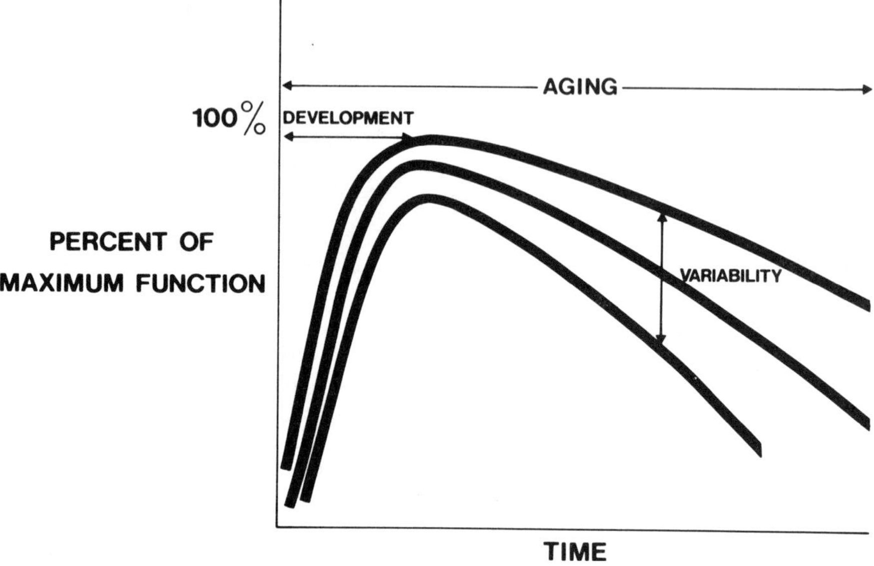

FIGURE 4-4 Function in relation to age.

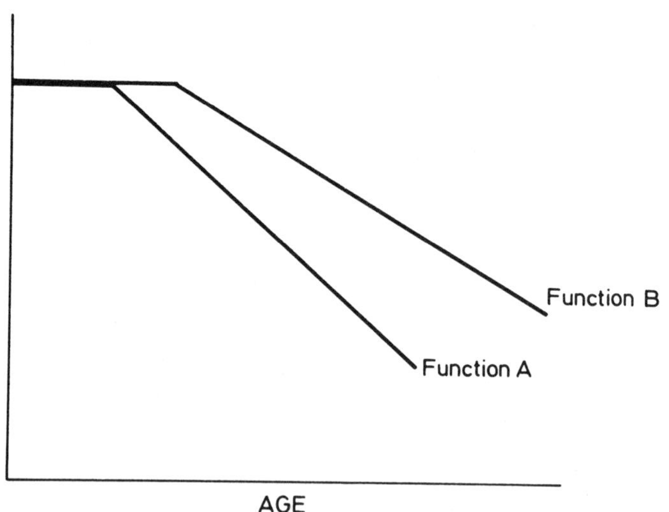

FIGURE 4-5 Differential function in relation to age.

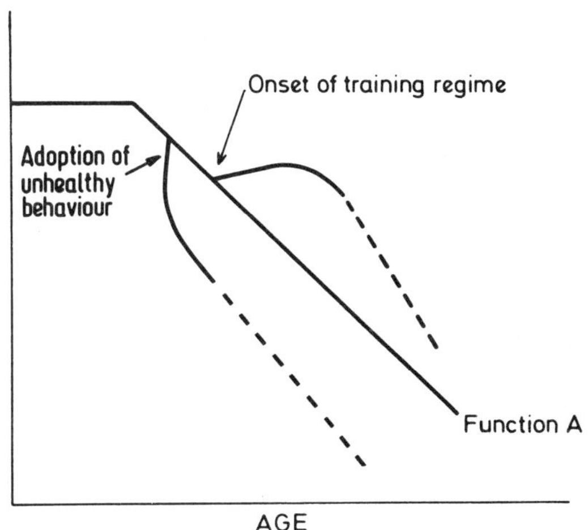

FIGURE 4-6 Function in relation to age and disease (modifying factors: healthy/unhealthy behavior).

training regimes for 3 months showed remarkable improvements in fitness, in muscle strength, and in cardiac responses to exercise (Anianson, Grimby, Rundgren, Svanborg, & Orlander, 1980).

Figure 4-7 illustrates the effect of acute disease on functioning. The effect may be a sudden and marked reduction in function. The long-term effect will be determined by the extent and nature of the disease and the effectiveness of treatment.

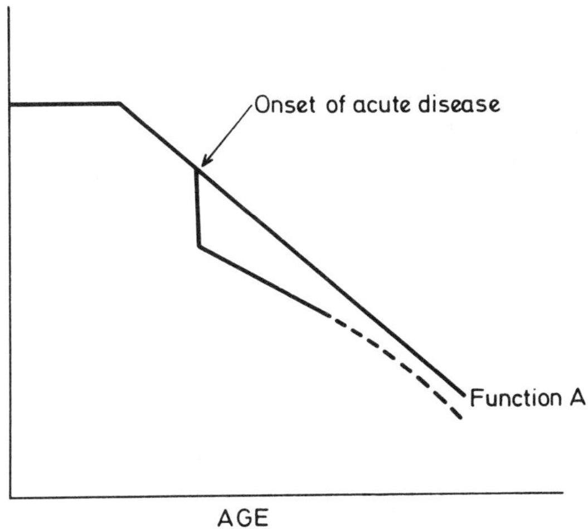

FIGURE 4-7 Function in relation to age (modifying factors: acute disease).

Figure 4-8 illustrates the effect of chronic disease on functioning. Chronic disease may produce a rapidly accelerating loss of function, but this may be mitigated by effective treatment and rehabilitation.

Cumulatively these simple diagrams suggest that the outcomes of aging in terms of function may be quite varied and complex because they are the product of the interplay of four factors: (1) heredity; (2) age changes; (3) disease (past and present); and (4) behavioral and environmental factors.

It has already been noted that medicine has tended to be concerned primarily or solely with the effects of disease. Such an approach can never be more than a partial success in dealing with the elderly.

Figure 4-9 is a simplified representation of the relationship between age and reduced functional capacity that identifies the probable distinctive relevance of geriatric medicine in very late life. This figure indicates that through early adulthood and into middle age most individuals possess "ample reserves." By early old age (65 for most individuals) reserves remain "generally adequate." Up to this point, the provision of medical care by the traditional system of primary care backed by specialists and subspecialists

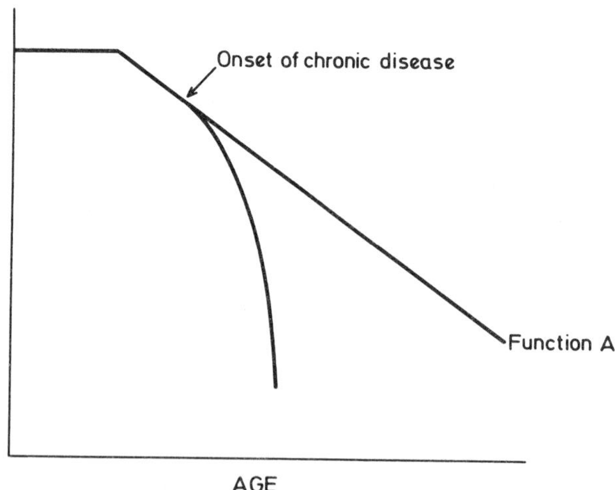

FIGURE 4-8 Function in relation to age (modifying factors: chronic disease).

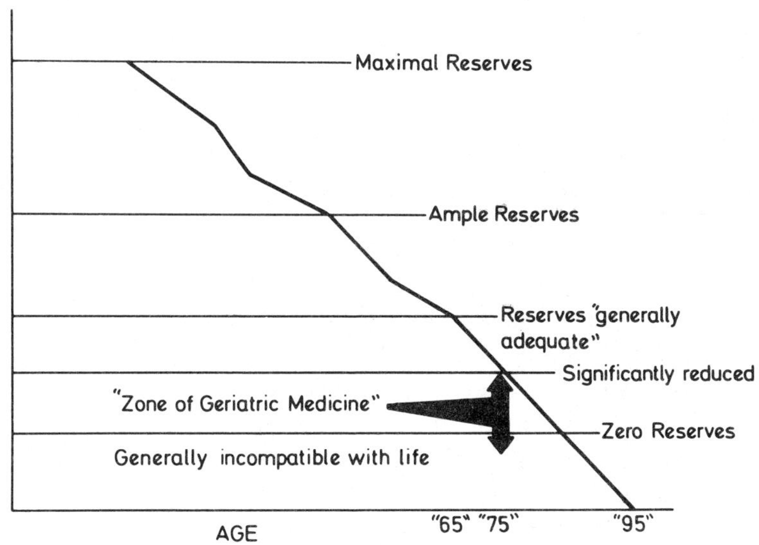

FIGURE 4-9 Function in relation to age and disease.

typically is adequate. But for those who survive into very old age (for most this means age 75), reserves may then become "significantly reduced." The rapidly increasing numbers of persons who survive into extreme old age are then moving through what I have termed the *Zone of Geriatric Medicine* and toward the theoretical state of "zero reserves." Persons who reach this last stage lead an increasingly precarious existence, in which any stress will produce a disproportionate disturbance, and any upset of homeostasis may be difficult (or even impossible) to correct. The outcome will vary:

1. Full recovery, which is most desirable at any age, is possible.
2. Death, for some the most desirable event if it comes swiftly and with dignity.
3. Survival, but at a much reduced level of independence so that the patient now needs constant nursing and frequent medical care. This is the least desirable outcome for the patient, the family, the professional attendants, and the general community.

A geriatric service has a special interest in all these outcomes, first in providing timely and expert care to ensure full recovery and maximum independence when possible; second, in arranging for suitable care where death is inevitable, with minimum distress and maximum dignity; and finally, where long-term hospital care is required, in arranging this care in the most appropriate and economical fashion.

Figure 4-10 illustrates the relationship between age and functioning, which adequate geriatric services are intended to promote. Maturity, following earlier rapid growth, is associated with a more prolonged maintenance of function than was previously believed possible; and senescence may be accompanied by a much more gradual decline in function than previously expected. These more favorable trends are followed by the sharp decline that occurs in the fourth phase of development, which I call *postsenescence.* Our understanding of these matters has been greatly enhanced by longitudinal studies, especially those conducted by Svanborg and colleagues in Gothenburg (e.g., Anianson et al., 1980). The start of this phase is indicated by the arrow in Figure 4-10. Phase 4 corresponds to my Zone of Geriatric Medicine. This is not to be confused with a terminal state, in which death is

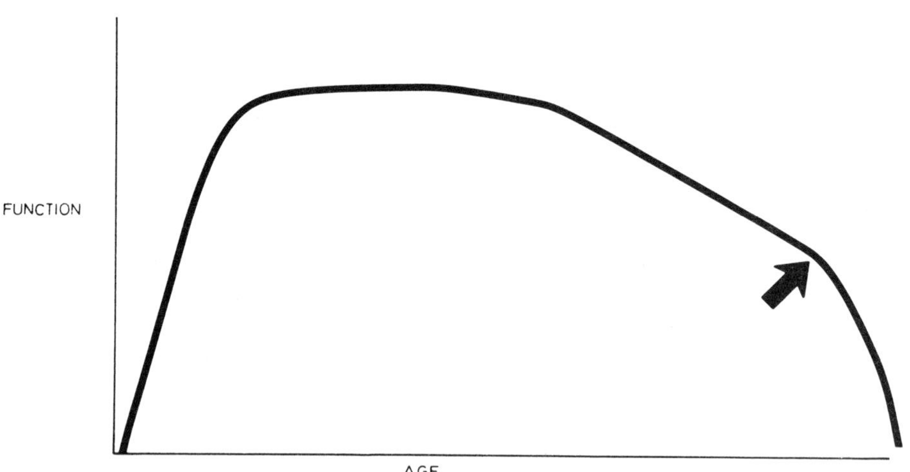

FIGURE 4-10 Function and age.

inevitable within a certain time. Although death in phase 4 is more likely to result from random and perhaps relatively minor stresses, patients may indeed survive for months or even years in this stage if they are able to avoid infections, injuries, or other stresses.

Demographic considerations that have already been alluded to dictate that increasing numbers of persons will survive into this postsenescence state—and this is one of the main arguments for a specialty of geriatric medicine to ensure the teamwork of medical and paramedical staff who are devoted to the special needs of postsenescent persons and thus provide optimum care for them. It has already been mentioned that age per se is not a sufficiently accurate criterion by which to judge when a person has reached this fourth phase of development, because so many other factors may be involved; however, it may be assumed that the dramatic (and continuing) increase in the 85+ group will result in increasing numbers of persons in this state. As has been pointed out, the medical needs of this group are different from those of young and middle-aged adults (and different also from those of the young old). Meeting these special needs is yet another justification for a specialty of geriatric medicine (in the same way that pediatrics sets out to understand and meet the needs of infants and young children).

This view of geriatric medicine is reflected in the definition Professor Alvar Svanborg and I proposed in a recent WHO document (World Health Organization, 1980): "Geriatric Medicine is that branch of medicine concerned with the special knowledge of symptomatology, the natural course of disease, treatment, rehabilitation and prevention in relation to patients in whom changes resulting from age contribute significantly to the clinical picture."

THE DEVELOPMENT OF GERIATRIC SERVICES IN THE UNITED KINGDOM

It is well known that specialization in geriatric medicine occurred earlier in the United Kingdom than in any other developed country, and, with all its faults and deficiencies, the UK system of health care for the elderly is probably better than that in any other country—it certainly provides better value for the money.

Several myths persist in relation to the United Kingdom system of care:

1. That it is the natural consequence of the National Health Service ("socialized medicine" in U.S. parlance). In fact, the ground rules were established long before the National Health Service was, and it was indeed already a thriving specialty in some areas.
2. That there is one monolithic pattern of geriatric care throughout the country. The truth is that there are many models—varying from age-related systems with high turnover that provide for all episodes of acute hospital care, to slow stream systems that emphasize rehabilitation and custodial care.

Thus, healthy argument and debate occur as to the proper role of geriatric medicine at present and in the future. The historical development of the specialty in Britain to this point has undergone three phases (Williamson, 1979).

Phase I

Phase I was the great personal triumph of Dr. Marjory Warren (Warren, 1943, 1946, 1948), whose leadership made three important contributions:

1. The conviction that no patient should ever be consigned to a chronic care facility without prior geriatric assessment and provision for rehabilitation (Williamson, 1981b). This has remained a golden rule of British geriatrics and must have saved countless thousands of elderly patients from inappropriate placement in long-stay institutions (Sheldon, 1971). It must also have saved the Health Service many millions of pounds in each year since its inception.
2. Dr. Warren's equally startling discovery that, in old age, rehabilitation was frequently successful (even in such unfashionable and unpromising conditions as stroke).

3. The discovery of the woeful ignorance of doctors and other health workers about the management of sick elderly patients.

This phase was soon succeeded by Phase II.

Phase II

The development of community services followed. Early in the evolution of the specialty it was discovered that preadmission visiting of referred patients made it possible to avoid inappropriate admission and to provide more appropriate alternative forms of care.

This led to two further developments:

1. The improvement in domiciliary and community services was inevitable as doctors of the caliber of Dr. Warren and her fellow pioneers entered the homes of the elderly and realized the true nature of the elderly's needs.
2. Day care/day hospitals and day centers were created.

Phase III

Then came the phase of preventive action and educational advances such as:

1. The documentation of unreported and unrecognized need among the elderly at home (Anderson & Cowan, 1955; Williamson et al., 1964).
2. The subsequent interest in case finding and earlier detection of stress among patients and those who care for them (Williamson, 1981b).
3. Increasing interest in education for doctors and other professionals in care of the elderly, and the foundation of the first Chair of Geriatric Medicine in Glasgow in 1965.

These three phases of development are now behind us and British geriatrics is moving into Phase IV. There exists considerable argument as to what Phase IV should consist of. In general, four options for the future have been proposed:

1. Abandon the specialty of geriatrics, leaving care of the elderly to general practitioners and internists who would seek help from subspecialists as required.
2. Develop an age-related specialty, as in pediatrics.
3. Integrate geriatrics with internal medicine, with the geriatrician being a full member of the acute-care team.
4. Preserve geriatric medicine as a full specialty, using a system of selective referral while pursuing policies aimed at realignment of geriatrics with mainstream medicine.

I shall now consider each of these options in some detail in the next section.

THE FUTURE OF GERIATRIC MEDICINE

Abandon the Specialty

This is a cry that has arisen from time to time since the earliest days of the specialty. Possibly the last despairing echoes in the United Kingdom were from Leonard in 1976 in an article titled "Can Geriatrics Survive?" The author's answer to his own question was a resounding negative, which he based mainly upon two deficiencies he identified and regarded as fatal flaws:

1. "Geriatrics has completely failed to attract enough staff."
2. "There are no clinical processes or techniques which are unique to geriatrics which is why the specialty is unattractive."

These criticisms were trenchantly posed but totally without supporting data.

Recruitment problems in geriatrics in the 1960s and 1970s were undoubtedly great. This problem, however, must be viewed in the context of the phenomenal expansion in the specialty. Thus, during the years 1966 to 1977 the mean increase in consultant establishment for all specialties was 34.3%, while for geriatrics it was almost three times as much (111.1%). Other "shortage specialties" were having their recruitment problems also, but their expansion was much less dramatic, for example, radiology (35.1%), anesthesiology (43.1%), and mental handicap (43.7%). The last shortage specialty, which was in fact the second most rapidly expanding, experienced 2½ times less growth than geriatrics. Even if geriatrics had been a most fashionable specialty, it might well have faced recruitment problems in light of such a phenomenal expansion. Far from being an attractive career, leadership in the specialty had problems in attracting young doctors who either had no experience of geriatric medicine or may actually have acquired highly negative impressions as a result of their clinical training (Gale & Livesley, 1974).

I believe that attacks of this nature upon the specialty often tell us more about the attackers than they do about geriatric medicine. Thus, it is not acceptable to attack elderly and geriatric patients, but it is always open season for shooting geriatricians. This sport has been by no means confined to the United Kingdom, and there are those in North America who continue to quote Leonard's paper despite the fact that no one wrote in support of the paper in the considerable correspondence published in the *British Medical Journal* following Leonard's article (Reichel, 1980).

As to the question of whether geriatric medicine possesses unique clinical processes or techniques, I am not at all convinced that these are the criteria by which the validity of a specialty ought to be judged. If pressed, I would suggest that our special skills in rehabilitation and in multidisciplinary teamworking mark us as separate and distinct from most other hospital specialties.

Adopt an Age-Related Model

This model has been widely promoted in England and Wales, but has found less favor in Scotland. It was originally advanced mainly as a means of improving recruitment to the specialty.

In this type of service the geriatric unit deals with all patients over a certain age requiring hospital care, usually those patients over 75 or over 65. Several descriptions of such services exist (e.g.,

Bagnall et al., 1977; O'Brien et al., 1973). There is no doubt that highly efficient geriatric services have been developed but I have some misgivings:

1. There tends to be an overemphasis in this model upon hospital care, and because 98% of the elderly are not in hospital, this yields an unbalanced and incomplete view.
2. If widely adopted, it would require massive shifts in resources from acute to geriatric services. This could exacerbate tensions between geriatricians and internists, and I cannot imagine its being widely tolerated in most developed countries.
3. It could lead to duplication of expensive equipment and highly trained staff as two parallel "acute" services evolved.
4. I cannot readily accept that debarring internists from treating all older patients can be in their long-term best interest—or that of the profession and general public. I fully accept that for many elderly patients the correct management is the same as for younger patients. For example the 75-year-old person with a circumscribed medical problem may be most appropriately dealt with by the family physician or internist.
5. The preoccupation with hospital care could distract the geriatrician from equally important aspects of geriatric medicine, such as prevention, community care, or support for carers. The importance of ensuring the geriatrician's interest in long-term care must also be stressed. After all, it was concern within this sector that led the pioneers to take an interest in care of the elderly.
6. I have an additional misgiving that this model has been devised more to suit the professional requirements of modern doctors rather than to meet the needs of patients and those responsible for their care.

There is one other point that has not, so far as I am aware, been brought out before. This relates to age-related services that use 75+ as the cut-off point. Such a policy may deny geriatric care to patients aged 65 to 74 who really ought to receive such care because their needs are geriatric. In order to investigate this point,

I have analyzed the referrals to my own department from general practitioners for 1983. Results are in Table 4-1.

This table shows that a substantial proportion of patients aged 65 to 74 had features that ought to direct them toward a geriatric service. Perhaps it is only necessary to point out that of all the frequently incontinent patients, almost one quarter were aged 65 to 74.

It is true that few age-related departments are operated with a rigid 75-year-old barrier; nevertheless, those departments with such an arrangement undoubtedly deny some geriatric patients the special care they need. At the same time, some patients in this age group (and a smaller proportion aged 75+) will find their way into a geriatric unit, even though their medical needs could be met adequately by the ordinary internal medicine service (or by their family physician).

Once again it is reiterated that age per se is not a good or reliable predictor of geriatric need, although it must be repeated

TABLE 4-1 GP Referrals to Geriatric Unit, City Hospital, 1983

	Age 65–74	Age 75+	Younger group as percentage of age of all referrals
Mobility			
Outdoors freely	37	76	34%
Indoors freely	53	203	21%
With mechanical aid	34	203	14%
With human aid	30	133	20%
Chair/bedfast	38	149	18%
Wheelchair	7	13	35%
Urinary incontinence			
No	141	537	21%
Occasional	28	150	16%
Frequent	21	68	24%
Catheterized	4	22	15%
Home help			
Yes	51	329	13%

that the rapid increase in the 85+ age group makes it certain that the numbers of those requiring a geriatric approach will increase rapidly.

Complete Integration with General Medicine

In this model of geriatric service, the geriatrician becomes a full member of the acute/internal medicine team and deals with patients of all ages while maintaining a special interest in older patients. This pattern has been promoted especially in Newcastle and Oxford (Evans, 1983).

I have the same reservations about this model as those I have outlined for the age-related model, particularly the equation of geriatric medicine with the clinical medicine of old age. This is unsatisfactory because it does not emphasize prevention and community care enough.

Another practical objection is that this integrated service arrangement ensures that old people go first into an acute medical ward, and thereafter the "geriatric patients" are transferred to the geriatric ward (called "rehabilitation ward" in Evans' report). Everyone with experience in these matters will know how relocation may upset these patients and retard (or prevent) their recovery. To arrange deliberately that such patients should experience not one but two relocations must be seen as unsatisfactory.

Further, doubts have been expressed about the ability of one individual doctor to cope with the whole range of adult medicine in addition to the considerable demands of geriatric medicine with its wide scope and range of activities. Doubtless there exist some latter-day Leonardo Da Vincis who possess this range of talents, but most of us will find ourselves fully taxed in coping with geriatric medicine alone.

The assertion is often made to support this model (as well as the age-related model) that by accepting a full range of acute care work, the geriatrician and related junior staff will enjoy greater work satisfaction, and therefore recruitment will improve. The corollary is usually left unstated, that is, that the rest of the work with the elderly is generally dull and uninteresting. This, of course, is what our pioneers were at such great pains to refute. Is it possible that some physicians who crave extra acute care are thus seeking to enhance their own self-esteem and that their original commitment to geriatrics was in fact a second best? One can only speculate upon the existence and motivation of such reluctant geriatricians.

Selected Referral Pattern to a Geriatric Service

In this model the geriatric service sets out to offer help to those who have been selected as needing a specialized kind of care, that is, those with multiple medical, social, and rehabilitation needs, especially those who are within (or approaching) the Zone of Geriatric Medicine discussed above. In this way, the geriatric service does not seek to compete for the acute care of old people who have a single illness or those with circumscribed clinical needs who ought to be managed by the family physician or internist.

Selection is usually by the general practitioner, who soon will learn the type of patient to refer to the geriatric service. Even if general practitioners are untutored in these matters, the arrival of an active geriatric service in their midst will soon make them aware of selection criteria.

This approach, which I favor, has many advantages:

1. The special identity of geriatric medicine is protected against submergence within internal medicine.
2. Correct emphasis is placed upon the special needs of geriatric patients irrespective of age.
3. Due attention can be paid to age and behavioral factors as well as to traditional pathological diagnosis.
4. Emphasis is placed upon prevention, including protection of carers against excessive demands.
5. If combined with deliberate policies of offering a geriatric contribution to other specialties, this model brings the specialty back into the mainstream of medicine. Geriatrics can then be practiced in full partnership and not as a "poor relation" to other specialties such as internal medicine,

orthopedic surgery, psychiatry, and emergency medicine (Barker et al., 1985; Burley et al., 1979, 1984).

This selected referral system thus ensures that the majority of geriatric patients are referred initially to the geriatric service. For those who appear first in other settings either from incorrect referral or other cause, the geriatric service provides a safety net into which they will eventually fall and thus receive the benefits of geriatric skill and knowledge.

The effectiveness of the contribution of geriatrics to acute medical wards has been fully described (Burley et al., 1979). This involvement resulted in marked reduction in mean stay of elderly patients in the acute wards (e.g., females aged 65+ had their mean stay reduced from 26 to 17 days, and for women aged 85+ the figures were 49 and 22 days). This was achieved by more rapid discharge to home, and not by more frequent transfer to the geriatric unit. A recent U.S. publication (Barker et al., 1985) showed how the adoption of this concept of geriatric consultation within acute hospitals leads to a significant reduction in prolonged stay in acute hospitals for patients aged 70+.

Similar benefits (although not similarly quantified) have accrued to orthopedic surgery through the contribution from one of my senior colleagues. This has been described elsewhere (Burley et al., 1984). Patients are seen in the acute orthopedic department, and advice is offered on their medical conditions. For those who require it, there is rapid transfer to a combined geriatric-orthopedic rehabilitation unit where the joint approach has proved very successful.

There are various methods of cooperating with geriatric psychiatry, but regular meetings and frequent consultations in each other's wards and in day hospitals with joint case conferences can usually be readily arranged. This will often lead to other more formal and closer means of collaboration. Somewhat belatedly, in Edinburgh we have started to take into our service geriatric patients from the accident and emergency department of the largest hospital in the area. Once again, this is a method of helping to salvage those geriatric patients who have slipped through the net of the selective referral system.

The Achievement of a Selected Referral Service

It has been implied (especially by age-related model enthusiasts) that the selected referral type of service tends to result in slow turnover and waiting lists. In order to refute this, I shall present some statistics and results from my own department of geriatrics.

The patient, having been referred by the general practitioner, is visited at home by a physician from the geriatric service. This practice was initially established in the days when we still struggled to cope with waiting lists, and hence new referrals had to be seen prior to admission in order to allocate priority. There has been no waiting list since this unit opened 9 years ago, and yet we still prefer to visit in this way. We did an analysis of the benefits of this practice (Arcand & Williamson, 1981) that showed that an adequate initial clinical assessment was almost always readily achieved while a very large amount of paraclinical information was also obtained. This ranged from vital information about current medication, accident hazards in the home, and evidence of self-neglect, to the detection of actual or threatened exhaustion in a key carer. In addition to these advantages, we felt that seeing how the old person functioned in his or her own home environment was much more relevant than functioning observed as an outpatient, in an emergency room, or in a hospital ward. The patient certainly is given the chance to "take on the system" on the patient's own terms rather than on the doctor's. An extra-important benefit of home visiting is that it enables the geriatric service to respond very rapidly and yet keep open all options for future management. Thus two thirds of patients are seen within 3 hours of referral, and 90% on the same day. This enables us to put into practice what we preach, namely, that *all* need in old age is a matter of urgency, no matter what the underlying pathology may be.

Figure 4-11 shows the outcome of the home visits. For example, 37% of general practitioner referrals were admitted to the geriatric unit, and 60% were dealt with in some other way by the geriatric service. It should be noted that 5% eventually required long-term care, either extended care or nursing home care. The mean stay in the geriatric assessment ward is 19 days, which is only 1 day more than that in the integrated service described by Evans (1983). There is no waiting list for admission. The 3% admitted to another hospital represents those who are judged to require other forms of care (e.g., cardiac pacemaker) or the small minority who are seen by us and who require immediate admission, but for whom we have no available bed. This is our failure rate, but even in these cases if they are "genuinely geriatric" we will try to take them over within a few days or at the earliest opportunity; certainly so if the patient is already known to our department.

The rapidity of response is illustrated in Figure 4-12, which shows the interval between referral and admission for the 37% who are admitted. Note that 70% are admitted on the day of referral and 21% the next day, that is, 91% within 24 hours. This speedy response enables us to deal with acutely ill patients—not

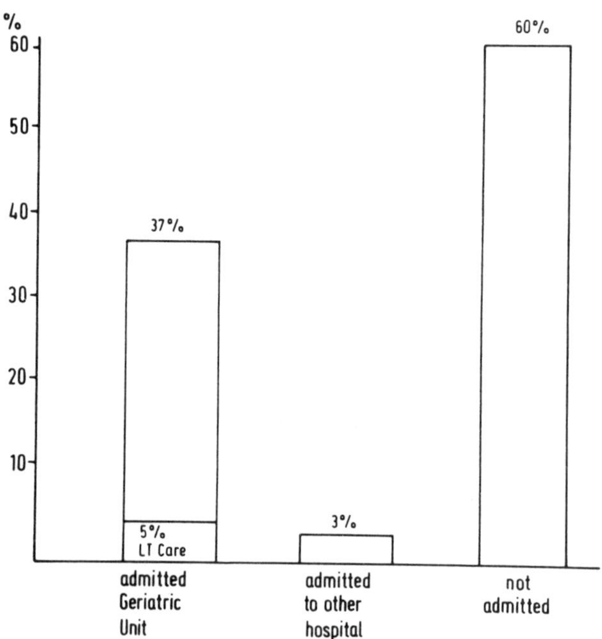

FIGURE 4-11 Proportion of patients referred by GPs: admitted and not admitted.

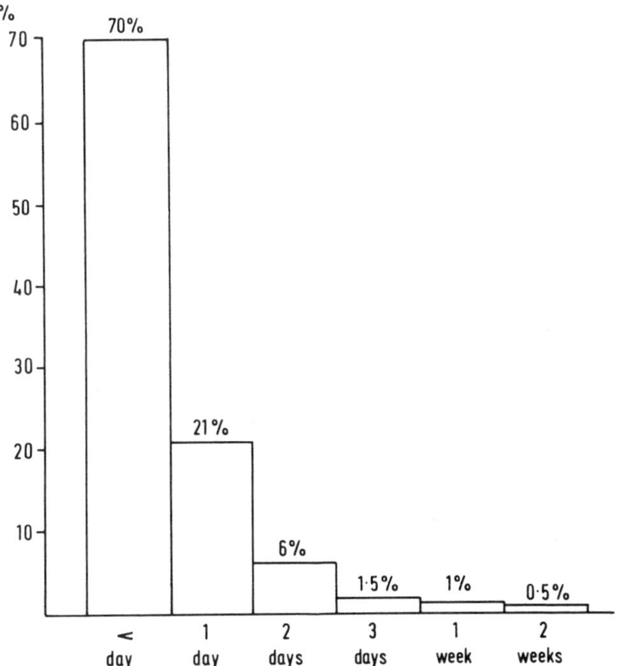

FIGURE 4-12 GP referrals: Interval from referral to admission to assessment unit.

because there is acute illness but because that illness is occurring in a geriatric patient.

Figure 4-13 indicated the outcome of patients who are not admitted to the geriatric wards. The largest proportion by far were admitted to our geriatric day hospital. This facility has been fully described as an integral part of our comprehensive geriatric service (Morales et al., 1984). Once again, there are no waiting lists for enrollment in the day hospital, most arriving there within 24 to 72 hours of first being seen.

The next most common service is advice only to general practitioners who increasingly seek our advice about optimum management of their elderly patients. It will be observed that 11% are assigned for respite admission. This may mean a straight "holiday admission" to enable families to have a well-earned break, but in-

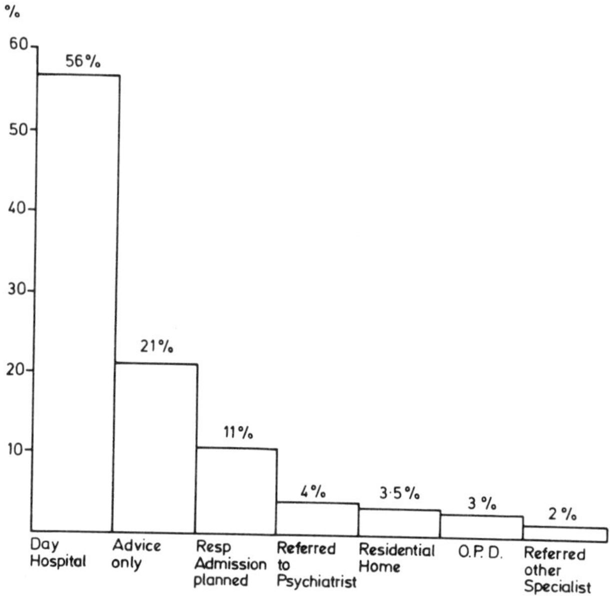

FIGURE 4-13 Action taken for patients referred by GPs *not* admitted to unit.

creasingly respite admissions are part of a system of shared care in which the geriatric service offers to look after the elderly person on a planned and regular basis. We have no doubt that this arrangement enables many families to go on supporting elders for very much longer than they would be able to do without this help. It is noteworthy that in more than a quarter of a century of this activity I cannot recall a single instance in which families have failed to honor a respite agreement by receiving the patient back in the planned fashion.

Figure 4-13 also shows that we do not request large numbers of consultations from other specialists. Only 2% are referred to another discipline. Probably the 4% referred for psychiatric opinion is too low because our local psychogeriatric service still struggles to cope with inadequate resources, in terms of staff as well as other items. Fortunately, this service is now improving and expanding.

Figure 4-14 shows the outcome for patients who are admitted to the geriatric assessment unit. Note that 70% are discharged, 16%

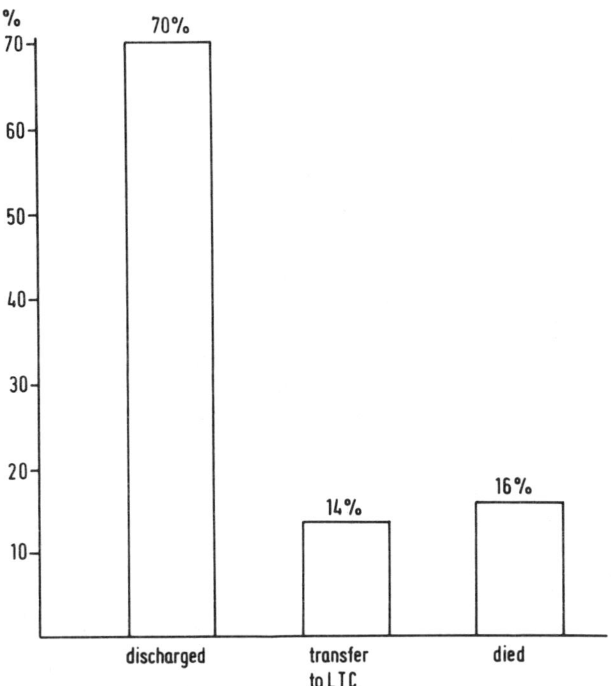

FIGURE 4-14 Outcome for patients admitted to assessment wards.

die within 3 months, and 14% require continuing institutional care. Such care almost always is provided within the 180 continuing care beds of our geriatric service.

The relatively high discharge rate has special significance and implies a high readmission rate. It might be claimed that to boast of a high readmission rate is somewhat perverse. But reflection will indicate that we are merely accepting and responding appropriately to the often rapidly changing needs of geriatric patients. Our aim is to provide an immediate and flexible response to these changes so that the patient is guaranteed readmission when circumstances so indicate. Thus we seek to have the patient in the hospital when necessary and in the community whenever fitness permits. In this way many elderly and aged patients spend 1 to 3 weeks in our wards several times per year for the final few years of their lives. They prefer it this way and so do we.

CONCLUSION

I have reviewed the nature of need in old age and have indicated that there is an increasing number of aged persons who require a specialist geriatric approach. I have described the true nature of need in old age and discussed the different patterns of geriatric care developed in the United Kingdom to meet these needs.

I have favored the so-called selective referral service, which I believe retains the best features of the British tradition of geriatric care. I believe that this pattern of geriatric service can readily be transplanted into other health care systems because it offers appropriate care for geriatric patients without threatening other specialists and disciplines. On the contrary, a generous offer of geriatric support for other relevant specialties will improve the image of the specialty and make it acceptable within the mainstream of medicine.

It has been alleged that geriatricians are merely usurping the general practitioner's function, but we would refute this, and the following response from our GP colleagues strongly suggests that they too see our efforts as complementing their own (Table 4-2).

The development of a specialist geriatric service has been the response to the marked aging of the population in the United Kingdom. The question must be asked: "Can any of this experience be applied within other countries with different health care arrangements?"

Applicability of United Kingdom Models of Geriatric Care to North America

It is obvious that the health care of the elderly in any country must be developed in line with past and present traditions, and must

TABLE 4-2 General Practitioners' Views

Do you find the geriatric service satisfactory?	99% Yes
Do you find the unit's practice of home visiting to be beneficial	
to patients?	99% Yes
to carers?	100% Yes
to general practitioners?	98% Yes

(Anonymous questionnaire sent to 80 general practitioners; 94% response)

also be acceptable to the public (including the elderly) and to the professions involved. Any system must also provide good value for the money. In this context, it is well known that the system of geriatric care in the U.S., which relies to a large degree upon acute care plus nursing home provision, is associated with accelerating costs that cannot be sustained in the future. Hence, some change is going to be necessary. I would recommend that some form of specialty geriatric service should be developed based upon the selected referral model described in this chapter.

Several points require emphasis:

1. As I have argued above, some old people have special needs and therefore require a special approach. I cannot see how these complex needs can be met without the enthusiastic and dedicated efforts of multidisciplinary teams who elect to specialize in this field. I read with great interest the excellent Beeson Report (Institute of Medicine [IOM], 1978) and fully appreciate that in 1978 it might not have been politic to recommend the establishment of a formal practice specialty in geriatrics, especially in view of the prevailing and commendable climate of opinion against further subspecialization in medicine. However, it should be appreciated that geriatric medicine is not just one more subspecialty. It is indeed a different way of practicing medicine that demands some new ideas and knowledge combined with the rediscovery of older and previously valued forms of practice, such as the house call as the optimum way of initiating geriatric care in many instances.
2. The great importance of providing a team approach must be accepted. The comprehensive assessment of need in old age cannot be based upon a traditional pathological diagnosis, but rather requires the skills of the nurse, the therapist, and of the social worker—not operating as separate professions, but acting together in a true team fashion.
3. Some mechanism must be provided to ensure that the full range of services will be available as the need is identified. This implies also that resources are provided in a balanced fashion and effectively coordinated. This, as has been argued above, is the natural function of a geriatric service, and in its

absence balance and coordination may not occur at all or may do so only haphazardly.

4. Services must be available to patients and carers according to their need and not according to their ability to pay. The system in the U.S. offers financial support for medical procedures (diagnostic and therapeutic), but often fails to provide support for items that are equally important in enabling the old person to remain at home (by provision of homemaker service) or for the family carers to continue their supporting role (by planned respite admissions and by good day care facilities). Although the notion that families ought to be self-sufficient in care of their aged members may be in line with the American ethic of rugged independence, it is an inadequate and costly approach to care for the elderly in any modern society. All our experience leads us to the conclusion that families who are offered prompt and timely help with a guarantee of continued support will continue their caring roles, whereas those who are denied such support may falter and fail as they are stretched beyond their limits of tolerance. Once breakdown of support has occurred, it is often irreparable and then may be presented as "family rejection" (MacMillan, 1960).
5. I have offered the selected referral model of geriatric care as being the best option for other countries, and I believe that it may be most readily adapted (at least in part) to other health care systems. It aims to provide specialized geriatric care for those who need it while leaving the "straightforward" clinical medicine of older patients to family physicians, internists, and other specialists. At the same time, it offers appropriate help to other disciplines as outlined above, always concentrating upon the true geriatric patient. I am aware that there may be no one analogous to the United Kingdom general practitioner who makes the appropriate selection in the first place, thus acting as a "gatekeeper" by allowing the true geriatric patient to proceed into the geriatric service while steering the others in another direction. Who is to be the gatekeeper in any such system developed in North America? I see no reason why this should not be the function of

several persons, such as any primary medical provider, whether family physician or internist. At present these physicians see patients who consult them first, but who then may be referred to another specialist. Is there any reason why, if such primary carers were fully acquainted with the function of a good geriatric service, they could not make appropriate referrals as do U.K. general practitioners? Likewise community nurses, nurse practitioners, and certain social workers might make referrals of patients and families whom they encounter in their daily work. It has already been outlined how referrals from internal medicine, orthopedics, and psychiatry can lead to more appropriate care and better use of resources.

6. In many respects, one of the most perplexing and frustrating aspects of medical care in the U.S. as seen by an outsider is the system of financial support, especially as it relates to medical remuneration. Much of this is based upon payment for items of service or for medical procedures, and because geriatric medicine is patient/family/community-oriented rather than based upon procedures, it is generally an inappropriate way of remunerating doctors for work with the elderly. Although a salaried service may seem incompatible with the entrepreneurial instincts of American medicine, it is by no means unpracticable, and there are now successful precedents upon which to build. I find it difficult to accept that sufficient doctors could not adapt to this change if it offered them the opportunity to contribute in a much more effective fashion to the needs of an aging population.

SUMMARY

The history of the United Kingdom specialty of geriatric medicine is a fascinating one and illustrates the potential benefits of having a pragmatic approach in which different methods have been tried and either developed or rejected according to outcome. Our successes and failures are worthy of close study by those in other countries also facing the geriatric explosion.

One thing is certain, and that is that any successful system of health care for the elderly must be based upon accurate and scientific study of their true needs—and this is what I have attempted to present here. Any attempt to force old people into inappropriate systems of care is bound to fail; hence the plea for a special approach tailored to the needs of aging persons and their carers.

I have little doubt that the great strength and innovative energy of North American medicine, freed of the shackles of inappropriate systems of care, will rise successfully to these new challenges. It must be emphasized, however, that there is no time to lose. Some fundamental rethinking of professional attitudes is now an urgent necessity.

REFERENCES

Anderson, W. F., & Cowan, N. R. (1955). A consultative health centre for older people: The Rutherglen experiment. *Lancet, 2,* 239.

Anianson, A., Grimby, G., Rundgren, A., Svanborg, A., & Orlander, J. (1980). Physical training in older men. *Age and Ageing, 9,* 186–187.

Arcand, M., & Williamson, J. (1981). An evaluation of home visiting by physicians in geriatric medicine. *British Medical Journal, 238,* 718–720.

Bagnall, W. E., Datta, S. R., Knox, J., & Horrocks, P. (1977). Geriatric medicine in Hull: A comprehensive service. *British Medical Journal, 2,* 102–104.

Barker, W. H., Williams, T. F., Zimmer, J. G., Van Buren, C., Vincent, S. J., & Pickrel, S. G. (1985). Geriatric consultation teams in acute hospitals. Impact on back-up of elderly patients. *Journal of the American Geriatrics Society, 33*(6), 422–428.

Burley, L. E., Currie, C. T., Smith, R. G., & Williamson, J. (1979). Contribution from geriatric medicine within acute medical wards. *British Medical Journal, 2,* 90–92.

Burley, L. E., Scorgie, R. E., Currie, C. T., Smith, R. G., & Williamson, J. (1984). The joint geriatric orthopaedic service in South Edinburgh, Nov. 1979 to Oct. 1980. *Health Bulletin, 42*(3), 133–140.

Evans, J G. (1983). Integration of geriatric with general medical services in Newcastle. *Lancet, i,* 1430–1433.

Gale, J., & Livesley, B. (1974). Attitudes toward geriatrics: A report of the King's Survey. *Age and Ageing, 3,* 49–53.

Institute of Medicine (IOM). (1978). *Aging and medical education.* Washington, D.C.: National Academy of Sciences.

Leonard, J. C. (1976). Can geriatrics survive? *British Medical Journal, i,* 1335–1336.

MacMillan, D. (1960). Preventive geriatrics. *Lancet, 2,* 1439–1441.

Morales, F. M., Carpenter, A. J., & Williamson, J. (1984). Dynamics of a geriatric day hospital. *Age and Ageing, 13,* 34–41.

Myers, G. (1985). Aging and worldwide population changes. In R. Binstock & E. Shanas (Eds.), *Handbook of aging and the social sciences* (pp. 173–198). New York: Van Nostrand Reinhold.

O'Brien, T. D., Joshi, D. M., & Warren, E. W. (1973). No apology for geriatrics. *British Medical Journal, 4,* 277–280.

Reichel, W. (1980). Is there a shortage of geriatricians? *New England Journal of Medicine, 303,*(15), 887.

Sheldon, J. H. (1971). Warehousing of the elderly. A history of British geriatrics. *Modern Geriatrics, 1,* 457–464.

Warren, M. W. (1943). Care of the chronic sick—A case for treating chronic sick in blocks in a general hospital. *British Medical Journal, 2,* 822–823.

Warren, M. W. (1946). Care of the chronic aged sick. *Lancet, i,* 841–843.

Warren, M. W. (1948). The evolution of a geriatric unit from a public assistance institution 1935–1947. *Proceedings of the Royal Society of Medicine, 41,* 337–338.

Williamson, J. (1979). Notes on the historical development of Geriatric Medicine as a specialty. *Age and Ageing, 8,* 144–148.

Williamson, J. (1981a). The spectrum of care. In *Appropriate care for the elderly: Some problems* (Royal College of Physicians of Edinburgh Publication No. 54).

Williamson, J. (1981b). Screening, surveillance and case finding. In T. Arie (Ed.), *Health care of the elderly.* London: Croom Helm.

Williamson, J., Stokoe, I. H., Gray, S., Fisher, M., Smith, A., McGhee, A., & Stephenson, E. (1964). Old people at home: Their unreported needs. *Lancet, i,* 1117–1120.

World Health Organization. (1980). *Health care of the elderly: Implications for education and training of physicians and other health professionals.* Discussion Paper by A. Svanborg & J. Williamson. WHO EUR/HCE/10/1, February 1980.

5
Health Care for the Elderly: Canadian Experience

Malcolm G. Taylor

The friend of humanity cannot recognize a distinction between what is political and what is not. There is nothing that is not political. Everything is politics.

Thomas Mann, *The Magic Mountain*

Politics is but medicine writ large.

Rudolph Virchow

An examination of Canadian experience indicates that it is difficult to separate the distinctive role of the hospital in health care for the elderly from the changing role of the acute care hospital in general. It is also difficult to separate satisfactorily that changing role from other components of the health care system, because they too are undergoing changes that impact not only on themselves but on other components as well. Moreover, it is evident that these changes have been effected by political decisions based on publicly expressed demands, on a changing mix of professions and paraprofessions and their interests, on new technology, and on economic and political realities. In short, health care for the elderly cannot be divorced from the whole of the health care system; the health status of an elderly person may depend more on access to health services before the age of 65 than after. It is equally difficult to separate health care from income maintenance programs that might make the difference between independent living and institutional care. Nor can consideration of the political decisions that shape the system ignore that Canada is a federal state, with its jurisdiction divided in the field of health and social services with the provinces.

What I have attempted, therefore, is to put the main theme of this discussion of care for older adults in the perspective of a universal, comprehensive, government-administered health care system. Although some consideration is given to the emerging distinctive role of the hospital, my discussion may best be considered as background provided by the experience of Canada. I will leave the more highly specialized theme of medicine's views to my medical colleagues. Underlying this presentation and frequently manifested in the text is my belief that Thomas Mann and Rudolph Virchow were right: It is not love, but politics, that makes the world go round.

CANADIAN GOVERNANCE

Any discussion of the health care system in Canada is inevitably complex because we are a federal state with divided jurisdictions. There are three fundamental problems in any federated nation: (1) the initial division of powers between the central government and the constituent parts that alter over time through constitutional amendments and court interpretations; (2) the division of revenue sources between the two jurisdictions to meet their assigned responsibilities; and (3) the inevitable disparities among the provinces or states in the yields from any revenue source, with the resulting differences in their respective capacities to provide levels of service approaching national standards. Until World War II these disparities between the "have" and "have-not" provinces were glaring, but since then Canada has taken major steps to bolster the financial underpinnings of all the provinces to enable them to meet, among other demands, those of the three growth industries of our times—health, education, and social services. To this end, two major strategies have been employed by the federal government: transfer payments to the provinces and transfer payments to individuals and families.

Transfer payments to the provinces are of three kinds: (1) Over time the federal government has reduced its personal and corporation income tax rates, leaving this so-called tax room to the provinces. (2) Beginning in 1947, tax agreements that provide unconditional block grants (referred to as "equalization payments") to low-income provinces have been negotiated every 5 years. Under the 1982 agreements, six provinces receive varying per capita payments that bring their overall revenues to the national average. (3) The third type of transfer payment is the familiar device of the conditional grant-in-aid for specific programs that, though falling under provincial jurisdiction, are considered to be in the national interest. Health insurance is the outstanding example, although there are scores of others.

The second major strategy consists of a variety of transfer payments to individuals and families. The first of these is a program introduced in 1945 called Family Allowances, which pays to every mother, irrespective of income, an indexed monthly payment (in 1985 $32.00) on behalf of each child up to the age of 16—and to age 18 if the child remains in school.

The second universal program—and for our concerns here, the more important—is a noncontributory, indexed Old Age Security payment (in 1985 $276.50 a month). This amount may be increased on an income-test basis by what is known as the Guaranteed Income Supplement. If the recipient's spouse is between ages 60 and 65, there is available a Spouse's Allowance, also on an income-test basis. These two (or three) payments, which can total as much as $1,000 per month in federal funds, may also be supplemented by provincial contributions, especially for those living in high-rent metropolitan areas.

In addition to the universal program is the Canada Pension Plan

(CPP), to which employees contribute 1.8% of income matched by an equal contribution from employers. Self-employed persons contribute 3.6%. Quebec administers a similar pension plan for its residents, with some minor differences. The CPP monthly payment is currently $381.00. There are also available, of course, various private pension and insurance plans. Pension reform is a perennial issue before the Canadian Parliament, and a major overhaul, particularly in the private sector, is imminent.

There are other social assistance programs directed toward other members of society (the blind, disabled, single parents, etc.) that are administered by provincial governments and municipalities, and these are typically cost-shared by the federal government. But the income maintenance programs I have outlined provide an important foundation of support for the elderly. No one in Canada is satisfied with the proportion of elderly persons, especially women living alone, whose income falls below the so-called poverty line despite large programs of low-rental and individually subsidized housing. But, given what we know about the circular effects of poverty and illness, these various income-support programs contribute immeasurably to the independent living and physical and mental well-being of many of the elderly.

CANADIAN HEALTH SERVICES PROGRAMS

Under Canadian federal–provincial division of powers, the national government administers an array of national health programs: food and drug standards, physical fitness and sports, health promotion, international health obligations, and health services for the armed forces, veterans, and native peoples. The vast majority of personal health services, however—as well as regulation of health professions, professional education, hospitals, and other health institutions—are jealously guarded provincial responsibilities. But the blanket power of the federal government to spend, even in areas of provincial jurisdiction, has dramatically reshaped Canadian health financing and delivery systems.

In 1945, the same year in which President Truman's health insurance proposals were being debated in the U.S. Congress, the federal (Liberal) government of Canada had offered the provinces federal cost-sharing of a comprehensive range of medical, hospital, dental, drug, and diagnostic services at the 1945–1946 Dominion-Provincial Conference on Post-War Reconstruction. With the failure of the conference to reach agreement on taxation issues, the health proposals lay in limbo, despite Gallup polls indicating 80% support for a national program (Taylor, 1978).

By 1950, however, four provinces had introduced hospital insurance programs of varying scope. At the 1955 Federal-Provincial Conference, called to renegotiate the tax agreements expiring in 1957, these four provinces not only requested increased tax transfers but insisted also that the federal government fulfill its 1945 commitment to health insurance. Surprisingly, this demand was supported for the first time by the Conservative government of Ontario.

In response, in 1956 the federal government proposed that the first stage of a health insurance program providing benefits of hospital insurance and diagnostic services be introduced. The program became operative on July 1, 1958, and all provinces had signed agreements by 1960. Virtually the total population of Canada was entitled to unlimited days of hospital care that were medically necessary and, except in Alberta and British Columbia, without user fees.

The second stage was the introduction on July 1, 1968 of the Medical Care Insurance program, which all provinces had joined by 1971. Although there were minor differences in the two programs, in general the federal government undertook to contribute one half of the aggregate expenditures by the provinces for the prescribed benefits. In return for the federal contributions, the provincial programs were required to meet five conditions:

1. Universality of coverage: insured services must be available to all residents upon uniform terms and conditions;
2. Comprehensiveness of insured services: all basic medically necessary services of the hospital at the standard war level; medically necessary services of physicians and surgeons in office, home, or hospital;
3. Accessibility: that insured services be provided in a manner

that does not impede or preclude, either directly or indirectly, by charges or otherwise, reasonable access by entitled persons;

4. Portability: that a province make payments due in respect of costs of insured services rendered to its entitled residents while outside the province; and
5. Public administration: that the plan be administered and operated on a nonprofit basis by a public authority appointed or designated by the provincial government (Taylor, 1978).

Financing

The federal contribution is paid from the general revenues of Parliament; that is, there is no earmarked federal health insurance tax. Originally most provinces, simply following insurance company and Blue Cross practice, levied premiums. Gradually, however, these were abandoned by most provinces, and currently only three provinces collect premiums; even in these provinces, recipients of social assistance as well as all residents over 65 are exempt, and low-income persons are subsidized.

By the mid-1970s there was widespread consensus that the original conditional grant-in-aid system had two major flaws:

1. The provinces constantly complained about the inflexibility of the conditions, especially the administrative requirements under the Hospital Insurance Agreements. Moreover, they claimed that the system distorted provincial decision making and priorities in that in allocating budget resources, expenditures of physician and hospital services were "50-cent dollars," while all other health services had to be financed solely from provincial revenues or, as they said, with "100-cent dollars."

   There was one serendipitous outcome of the original hospital insurance agreements, however. Under the act, mental hospitals were excluded. But provincial administrators quickly realized that psychiatric units that were within general hospitals would be cost-shared. One result was to bring a large portion of psychiatric treatment into the mainstream of health care.

2. The second flaw was the federal government's concern that it had lost control of its health budget because it was committed to match whatever the provinces decided to spend in 50-cent dollars on the two programs.

Accordingly, in 1977 three changes were negotiated (Taylor, 1985).

1. The federal government reduced its income tax levy by 12.5%, leaving this vacated tax room for the provinces to occupy—which, of course, all of them did. The 12.5% was calculated to approximate one half of the federal contribution under the original formula.
2. The federal government continued its cash grant calculated to equal the other half of its contribution (based on its 1975–1976 payments) to be increased each year in accordance with increases in the gross national product (GNP), and therefore no longer geared to actual provincial health expenditures on medical and hospital services.
3. In addition, the federal government contributed a new Extended Health Care Services grant of approximately one-half billion dollars, also to be increased in accordance with annual increases in GNP. Although it was an unconditional grant, the intent was to enable provinces to extend their nursing home and home care health services.

Through the changes introduced in 1977, both parties largely gained their objectives. The federal government achieved control, or at least predictability, with respect to its health budget. The provinces gained the flexibility they desired, because the federal government financial contributions no longer had any steering effects on provincial decision making. At the same time, the provinces became solely responsible for annual increases in health spending that exceed increases in GNP. The effect of this is not clear, for most of the provinces had already begun to introduce restraints on health budgets.

These restraint measures were, however, only one manifestation of the ferment of new ideas about the entire spectrum of the health care system. There were a number of reasons for the new attitudes. The first was the sheer magnitude of the health expenditures as a proportion of total provincial budgets. By 1979–1980 health expenditures among the provinces averaged almost 30% of total provincial expenditures, ranging among the provinces from a low of 20.9% to a high of 34.2%. A second factor was a growing consensus that the introduction of hospital insurance first had resulted not only in excessive development of the institutional sector but had also "educated" Canadians and their physicians to prefer inpatient care to ambulatory care. A reinforcing third element was the unprecedented (and only partly planned) increase in the supply of physicians.

But one of the most influential forces was the publication in 1974 by the Minister of Health, the Hon. Marc Lalonde, of a monograph, *A New Perspective on the Health of Canadians* (Lalonde, 1974). The main contribution of the paper was to provide a conceptual framework for analysis and evaluation of the health field. It suggested that there were four elements in the health field: human biology, environment, lifestyle, and health care organization. Examining the causes of morbidity and mortality, and the expenditures made on health facilities, professional education, and the delivery of treatment services, the report concluded that Canada had undoubtedly overextended her health services organization to the neglect of biologic research, environmental protection, and concern with health-threatening lifestyles. It confirmed what many had sensed—that the outer limits of the contribution of the medical model to the general health status of the population had been reached, if not exceeded.

It has often been observed that although we understand and, indeed, frequently applaud the revolutions of the past, we never fully comprehend the revolution in which we are currently engaged. In the postwar period no other segment of Canadian society has been subject to such a degree of change as has the health sector, beginning with the technological revolution within medicine itself (Thomas, 1983). To these intrinsic changes were added the conflicting ideas, proposals, and demands of federal and provincial governments, as well as those between medical and hospital associations and provincial governments, those between hospital administrators and medical staffs, and those between the medical profession and other professions seeking a larger share of the health care turf.

However, in determining the objectives and policies of the health care system and in managing the allocation of resources, the provincial governments have certain advantages over the federal government, in that one agency in each province, the provincial ministry of health, has jurisdiction over three major functions:

1. It is the central planning agency responsible for approving the location and size of all hospitals and other health care facilities, their programs, and their equipment, usually on the advice of regional or district health councils and their own experts and technical advisory committees. As I understand it, this compares with the certificate-of-need process in the United States.
2. The ministry negotiates and approves the budget of all hospitals and negotiates the fee-for-service schedules with the respective provincial medical associations. In U.S. parlance, this means that all health care institutions are paid on a prospective budget basis.
3. The ministry is the disbursing agency; it pays hospitals on the basis of the annual budget, and pays the physicians mainly on the fee-for-service basis, although salary and sessional indemnity arrangements are not uncommon.

Behind these unified planning, control, and payment organizations stand, of course, the more powerful ministries of finance, dedicated (as in all other countries) to a policy of health cost containment.

Because there are no costs for collecting premiums in the seven provinces that fund their programs from general revenues, and because hospitals are paid in monthly or semimonthly installments of their approved budget, the overall administrative costs of the health insurance system are estimated at about 2%.

But there is one other internal political factor affecting decision making and administration within the provincial governments. We are all aware of the interrelatedness of health and social services. At the federal level, health and welfare programs are combined in one department, Health and Welfare Canada. But in the provincial governments, the sheer size of the health budget gives such extraordinary power to the health minister that the social services are invariably assigned to a separate ministry, with its own distinct bureaucracy, different rules and regulations, and, in some provinces, even different types of regional organization.

Yet another factor having a similar effect is the difference in ownership of long-term care facilities. In all provinces, acute- and chronic-care hospitals are publicly owned. A few, such as university hospitals, are owned by provincial governments, and the others are owned by municipal governments, religious orders, and voluntary associations incorporated under the respective provincial Societies Acts. All are nonprofit. On the other hand, a high proportion of nursing homes are privately owned and are operated for profit.

The ensuing complexity in providing long-term institutional care is well illustrated in Ontario. The for-profit nursing homes are under the jurisdiction of the ministry of health. But homes for the aged, owned by municipalities, and religious and other voluntary associations are nonprofit organizations under the jurisdiction of the ministry of social services. The problems of coordination are compounded (Metropolitan Toronto District Health Council, 1984).

The Elderly Population

For whom have we built this enormous health care establishment? Well, obviously for the entire population of Canada, which now approximates 25 million or, for comparative purposes, about one tenth that of the United States. But we are here concerned with the elderly and their growing numbers, both in absolute terms and as a proportion of the total population (Denton & Spencer, 1982, 1983).

In the census year 1981, those aged 65 and over represented 9.7% of the total population, or nearly 1 in 10 (Health and Welfare Canada, 1983). In comparison with the United States, England and Wales, France, and Sweden, this would suggest that Canada might be placed in the young-old category. Since the turn of the century the rate of growth of the elderly has been double that of the population generally. The rate of increase of those over 80 during that period has been even more spectacular (a total population of 451,000 persons in 1981) and the total is projected to double by 2021. Or, to put it in more immediate terms, the over-80 group now constitutes 19% of those 65 and over, and by 2001 will constitute almost a quarter of the elderly. It is obvious that we are rapidly approaching the middle-old and old-old stages. The impact on the need for health services is both obvious and ominous.

A further factor related to the well-being of the elderly is the difference in employment rates. During the decade of the 1970s, the work force increased by 40%, and the percentage of women in the work force by 70%; but the percentage of males over 65 declined by almost 1% and that of women by 0.6%, undoubtedly due in part to a general practice of compulsory retirement at age 65. I might say, parenthetically, that under the Charter of Rights, which came into effect in April of 1985 as a result of amendments to our Constitution in 1982, discrimination on the basis of age is prohibited. This may mean an end to mandatory retirement at 65. Two provinces have already passed legislation prohibiting the practice. The effects are yet to be seen.

Future Implications

The magnitude of the combination of the three forces that drive the demand for health services—an increasing population, a rapidly shifting demographic profile, and already-high rates of utilization and institutionalization—have resulted in a flood of studies and reports by Statistics Canada (1982, 1984), Health and Welfare Canada, government commissions and task forces, and by independent academics. The most recent of these, one that draws on many of the others, is the report of a blue-ribbon Task Force on the Allocation of Health Resources, funded by the Canadian Medical Association (CMA, 1984). Obviously concerned with countering the charges of probable bias with which its appointment was greeted, the Task Force appointed a prestigious management consulting firm, Woods Gordon, to conduct the demographic and financial analyses. Their demographic projections are close to those I have already quoted. (For a parallel analysis on Ontario, see Gross & Schwenger, 1981; Ontario Council of Health, 1978.)

The analysts then projected the future percentage increases in health services utilization based solely on the demographic changes, assuming there would be no changes in the status quo organization of the health care delivery system. The highlights of this projection are: a required 64% increase in home care nurses, a 63% increase in long-term facilities, a 44% increase in acute care facilities, and a 28% increase in the supply of physicians over the current 20-year period (see, e.g., Metropolitan Toronto District Health Council, 1984).

The financial implications of the indicated increased utilization from demographic factors alone are astronomical, involving, by 2021, an increase in annual operating costs (in 1981 dollars) of 75%. The capital costs would be commensurate; the projected increased requirements for long-term facilities alone would involve construction of at least 1,000 300-bed facilities in the 40-year period. As the report stated, to follow our current course, "the costs will not only be prohibitive, [but] we will perpetuate the callous practice of warehousing the elderly."

The chief recommendation of the Task Force was deinstitutionalization, the adoption of policies that would reduce the proportion of the elderly who are in hospitals, nursing homes, and homes for the aged by a massive expansion of community resources. This brings us to the heart of the problem of meeting the growing needs of an increasingly elderly population—what might be encapsulated in the phrase "the politics of health care."

THE POLITICS OF HEALTH CARE

The health care political arena is both large and complex, and it is characterized by a high degree of government involvement and by an extraordinary array of interest groups representing both providers and consumers. The provincial medical associations have expanded their staffs of economists and public relations personnel, and they employ expert labor lawyers in their annual negotiations of the fee schedules. The medical associations have focused their efforts mainly on economic issues and on professional autonomy, including the right of the physician to deal directly with the patient regarding payment of the fee (which would encompass as well the right to extra-bill or balance-bill the patient beyond the fee set by the negotiated contract). The hospital and nursing associations have similarly expanded their research staffs but have placed less emphasis on economic issues and more emphasis on the direction the health system as a whole should take in promoting and maintaining health.

The major consumer organization is called the National Health Coalition, with counterpart organizations in most of the provinces. It is an umbrella organization of some 30 interest groups, including labor, teachers, nurses, and church groups. There are also scores, if not hundreds, of special-interest groups representing those afflicted with specific diseases. In addition to these groups—pressing their claims on government and urging changes in public policy—there is a host of academics, think tanks, and media commentators arguing in support of various strategies and policies.

At the center of this vortex is the Ministry of Health, acting on many issues in cooperation with the Ministry of Social Services, each with its network of advisory committees. All provinces, for example, have senior citizen advisory committees. Some provinces have endeavored to formalize interest-group participation through the establishment of health councils representing both providers and consumers. Further policy inputs come from standing legislative committees on health, as well as ad hoc committees appointed to consider specific issues. Opposition parties raise issues and propose alternative policies in the daily question periods and in debates on health matters in the legislatures or in Parliament.

The health ministries themselves have gone through an interesting metamorphosis. As late as the 1950s, every deputy minister of health in Canada was a medical doctor. But with the massive increase in health department budgets, senior management positions have been taken over by accountants, economists, and MBAs. At the present time, of the 11 deputy ministers of health, only 2 have medical degrees. The impact on public policy of this change in management personnel has not been assessed and may not be measurable.

But there is no doubt about the impact of the public debates on health care issues. No other policy issue rivals that of health in amount of public and media attention. The power of public opinion is well illustrated by the amendments to the Medical Care Act embodied in the Canada Health Act passed in 1984. Since the introduction of medical care insurance in 1968, the most festering issue has been the right of a physician to extra-bill or to balance-bill selected patients. The practice is defended not only by the medical associations (as the foundation stone of an autonomous profession) but also by, in particular, the Conservative governments of Alberta and Ontario. In 1979, when the practice reached its peak in Alberta, Nova Scotia, and Ontario, the National Health Coalition mounted a massive publicity campaign against the practice on the grounds that it violated the principle of universal accessibility.

In 1980 the Health Services Review condemned the practice on the grounds that it would lead to a two-tier fee system, one tier for the rich and another for the poor (Health Services Review, 1980). The following year the Parliamentary Task Force on Federal Fiscal Relations proposed penalties on provinces that tolerated either extra billing by physicians or authorized user charges to hospitalized patients (Parliamentary Task Force, 1981).

Finally, in April 1984, the Canada Health Act was passed by unanimous vote in the House of Commons. It provides for a reduction in federal payments to a province by the aggregate amount of such charges occurring. For example, at the present time, the province of Ontario loses about $50 million annually, which is the estimated aggregate of extra-billing by about 13% of Ontario's physicians. By 1985, five more provinces had abolished the practice and the new government of Ontario had indicated that it would give such a measure high priority.

Since the late 1970s, the Canadian Medical Association (CMA) and its provincial divisions have mounted a massive publicity campaign, charging that the treatment system is seriously underfunded, stressing that Canada allocates about 2% less of her gross national product to health services than do other Western nations. Charges that the provinces were diverting federal health contributions to nonhealth purposes led to the appointment of the Health Services Review in 1979, which concluded that this was not the case (Health Services Review, 1980). In 1981, the Parliamentary Task Force referred to above also examined the issue of underfunding and concluded that the public interest would not be served by expanded funding of the treatment system, although there was a strong case for increasing expenditures on public health and community services (Parliamentary Task Force, 1981).

This rejection of its claim that the system was underfunded was the primary reason that the CMA decided to fund its own task force, already noted. In addition to its strong positive recommendations respective to the elderly, the task force addressed the issue of adequacy of funding. It examined the conflicting evidence and arguments presented in the briefs it had heard and concluded that "Canadians are fed up with the shell game in progress with the levels of funding. . . . we cannot assess the extent of existing deficiencies and because there is no guarantee that putting more money into the system is necessarily the best way of improving health, the Task Force cannot make a clear-cut recommendation" (Parliamentary Task Force, 1981). To resolve the issue, the Task Force recommended the appointment of a representative national health council, which would conduct studies and continuously monitor the system. The provincial governments and, indeed, the provincial medical associations reject this proposal on the grounds that it would infringe on provincial autonomy.

In retrospect, the introduction of hospital insurance in 1958 and medical care insurance in 1968 marked what might be called the high-water point of Canadians' acceptance of and commitment to the medical model, and I have referred to the ferment of ideas and proposals for alternative services and health-promotion strategies that, since the Lalonde 1974 report, have increasingly informed public discussion and government action. But it should be stressed that it is not an either/or proposition. The case is better stated in the following terms: Having created a world-class system of hospitals, health professions, and educational institutions, and having achieved a physician/population ratio of 1:538 (of whom more than half of the physicians are primary care practitioners), Canada must now develop the alternatives while preserving the high-quality treatment services.

The main problem now is not, therefore, one of philosophy or policy of priorities; it is, rather, that in a period of restrained revenues, the large inventory of hospitals and physicians constitute an almost intractable first-priority demand on provincial health budgets.

As I mentioned earlier, during the 1970s health expenditures kept pace with growth in GNP, hovering around 7% throughout the period. By 1982, the proportion had risen to 8.4% due mainly to a decline in the rate of growth of GNP in 1981 and 1982, rather than due to an increase in the rate of health spending. But within that period, institutional costs had increased from 3.3% of GNP in 1970 to 4.7% in 1982. Expenditures on physicians' service remained constant throughout the period at a rate of about 1.2% of GNP, even though physicians continued to have the highest average incomes among all professions. The result is that, no matter how enlightened the new emphasis is regarding health promotion and community services for the handicapped and elderly, budget constraints have prevented the more rapid development of the alternatives that health planners and health ministry officials believe are essential.

But it has been observed that genuine change is most likely under only two conditions: (1) when the budget is in a state of feast, or (2) when the budget is in a state of famine. Although, by world standards Canada cannot be said to be in a state of famine, at this point, ingenuity and change must occur if Canada is to meet the inexorable increase in the needs of the elderly.

In fact, given the budgetary restraints of the 1970s and 1980s, it is perhaps remarkable that Canadians have turned the system around to the degree that we have. In a report prepared by Health and Welfare Canada for the 1982 World Assembly on Aging, it takes 7 pages of the appendix simply to list the provincial health, social service, and income maintenance programs administered by the provincial governments (Health and Welfare Canada, 1982).

HEALTH AND WELFARE PROGRAMS

These programs vary from province to province in their stages of development, in the range of benefits available, and in the proportion of residents having access to them. But even a cursory listing is impressive. All provinces have a basic public health nursing service; all provinces but one have day-care services; all have home care and homemaker programs, although in some provinces the coverage is spotty; most have senior citizen centers, although, again, not in all communities; most have subsidized road and air ambulance services; a half dozen have hospital day centers; several have dental programs; all have pharmaceutical programs (some paying part and others the total costs of prescribed drugs); several pay part or all of the costs of prostheses. Social services, subsidized housing and transit, and tax exemptions also contribute to independent living.

It is more difficult to generalize about the distinctive role of the acute care hospitals in the continuum of care. The most serious problem is the shortage of geriatricians and gerontologists. But geriatric departments have been established, usually in one or two teaching hospitals in each major center, and are available as consultants to several other institutions. A second major step is the development of discharge planning committees that begin their assessment and placement planning with respect to appropriate patients shortly after their admittance. Health and Welfare Canada has issued an extensive series of booklets providing guidelines for the establishment in acute care general hospitals of specialized geriatric units, stroke services, rehabilitation medicine, diabetic day care, adult psychiatric services, day surgery, and palliative care.

Undoubtedly the outstanding example in Canada of facilities providing a continuum of care is the Baycrest Centre for Geriatric Care in Toronto. Several establishments provide different levels of care under the Baycrest umbrella. These include the Home for the Aged, which provides residential accommodation, nursing care, and special care for mentally impaired residents requiring nursing services for their daily needs. Baycrest (chronic care) Hospital provides a wide range of services including podiatry, dentistry, pharmacy, radiology, occupational therapy, and physiotherapy. Baycrest Terrace provides self-contained suites for elderly persons who require a minimum of assistance, including heavy cleaning, linen service, the main meal of the day, and 24-hour nursing service in emergencies that includes the outpatient services of Baycrest Hospital. There is also a day-care service providing a full day's activities for companionship, rehabilitation, and recreation. Five hundred volunteers work at the Baycrest Centre. As the Task Force on the Allocation of Health Care Resources concluded, "It is a model that could be adapted to a wider community" (CMA, 1984). What is particularly significant is that the medical director at Baycrest Centre is head of the Division of Geriatrics at the Mount Sinai acute care general hospital in downtown Toronto.

In Alberta, a number of acute care hospitals have on their grounds facilities including a lodge, nursing home, and auxiliary hospital, thus facilitating a similar continuum of care. This "campus approach" is widely acclaimed and, if and when additional resources become available, may be part of the wave of the future (Schonfield, 1975).

In British Columbia, a province-wide long-term care (LTC) program has been developed, providing nursing home, home nursing, and homemakers' services. Four short-term assessment and treatment centers provide both inpatient and day-care services. An outstanding feature of the program is the comprehensive data base now available for policy research purposes (R. J. Ham, personal communication, 1985).

In concluding this discussion of the Canadian health system, including the role of the hospital in care of the elderly, the comments of Thomas Mann and Rudoph Virchow respecting politics are constantly reinforced. The transfer of control of the system from producers to consumers was clearly a political revolution. Prior to the introduction of hospital and medical care insurance, the hospital associations controlled the policies and, therefore, the politics of Blue Cross. The medical associations controlled the policies and, therefore, the politics of the (Blue Shield) medical care prepayment plans. The introduction of the government programs switched the policy decision-making process from the private sector arena to the public sector arena. Not only did this make the system more responsive to public needs, but also the requirement of universal coverage brought to all citizens what the prepayment plans and insurance industry had been able to bring to less than 40% of our people.

The greatest beneficiaries are the poor and the elderly. No longer is a resident of Canada required to put cash or an insurance policy up front to obtain either medical or hospital care; the sole criterion is medical necessity. The ending of the fear of crippling medical and hospital bills is a boon beyond description, especially for the retired elderly.

The centralizing in a single agency of each province of planning, facilities approval, and payment to health care providers meant that, for the first time, one person—the Minister of Finance—is responsible for the aggregate allocation of resources to health care, and that one other person—the Minister of Health—is responsible for the allocation of those resources within the health services spectrum. This has resulted in a reduction of emphasis on acute care hospital facilities and in a gradual shift to services more appropriate to individual needs.

Although spokesmen for the medical association have criticized the system as being monopolistic ("one paymaster") and underfunded, the medical profession in general agrees with some but not all of the government policies. In a survey of opinions and attitudes of the medical profession in five provinces representing the five regions of Canada (which two colleagues and I conducted in 1983) one question asked of respondents was to rank 10 different policy proposals (Taylor, Stephenson, & Williams 1984). Expansion of chronic care facilities and of home care programs ranked 1st and 2nd, but HMOs and training of nurse practitioners ranked 9th and 10th respectively. The first two types of propositions would, of course, free up more acute care beds that are now occupied by long term care patients. This objective is clearly understandable, because the combination of restraint on acute care beds and the large increase in the number of physicians has reduced the acute care beds-to-physician ratio by 25% over the past 10 years (from an average of 4.4 beds per doctor to 3.3 beds per doctor).

The charges that the government monopoly is frequently arbitrary in its decisions are probably inevitable when dealing with what appears to be an infinite capacity of the population to utilize health services in the face of finite resources to finance them. The charges of arbitrariness are most frequently heard during government/profession negotiations over increases in the medical fee schedules and when ministries of health make decisions affecting the amount and location of high technology and of specialized units such as those for open-heart surgery. But, as I have indicated, the health departments are advised not only by their own experts but also by technical advisory committees on which the medical profession is represented. Ultimately, the decision makers are responsible to the legislatures and parliament and they, in turn, are responsible to the electorate for whom the health services programs exist.

The role of the hospital and its medical staff in the continuum of care for the elderly is a crucial one. But, as I have suggested, that continuum, in fact, begins even before a child's birth. It is too early for us to judge what universal accessibility to medical and other health measures throughout the individual's lifetime will have during the post-65 stage. Many of the elderly who are now in long term care facilities or are receiving home care services have suffered the deprivations of 10 years of depression and 6 years of war. The approaching cohort of the elderly will be better educated, more affluent, and healthier. With the current enlightened leadership of the Canadian Hospital Association, of the Canadian Nurses Association, and of many leaders in the medical profession, I am confident that through their work with officials in the health ministries who are now inspired by the nature and magnitude of the challenge ahead, politics or the political process will ensure that the continuum of needs of the elderly will be met.

REFERENCES

Canadian Medical Association. (1984). *Health: A need for redirection.* Ottawa, Canada: Author.

Denton, F. T., & Spencer, B. G. (1982). *Population aging and future health care costs in Canada* (Research Report No. 35). Hamilton, Ontario, Canada:

McMaster University, Program for Quantitative Research in Economics and Population.

Denton, F. T., & Spencer, B. G. (1983). *The sensitivity of health-care costs to changes in population age structure* (Research Report No. 74). Hamilton, Ontario, Canada: McMaster University, Program for Quantitative Studies in Economics and Population.

Gross, M. J., & Schwenger, C. W. (1981). *Health care costs for the elderly in Ontario: 1976–2026* (Occasional Paper 11). Toronto, Ontario, Canada: Economic Council of Ontario.

Health and Welfare Canada. (1982). *Canadian government report on aging.* Ottawa, Canada: Department of Supply and Services.

Health and Welfare Canada. (1983). *Fact book on aging in Canada: Second conference on aging in Canada.* Ottawa, Canada: Department of Supply and Services.

Health Services Review. (1980). *Canada's national–provincial health program for the 1980's.* Ottawa, Canada: Health and Welfare Canada.

Lalonde, M. (1974). *A new perspective on the health of Canadians.* Ottawa, Canada: Health and Welfare Canada.

Metropolitan Toronto District Health Council. (1984). *Coordination of long term services in metropolitan Toronto.* Toronto, Ontario, Canada: Author.

Ontario Council of Health. (1978). *Health care for the aged.* Toronto, Ontario, Canada: Author.

Parliamentary Task Force on Federal–Provincial Fiscal Relations. (1981). *Fiscal federalism in Canada.* Ottawa, Canada: Department of Supply and Services.

Schonfield, A.E.D. (1975). *Alternatives to institutionalization for seniors.* Calgary, Alberta, Canada: University of Calgary, Department of Psychology.

Statistics Canada. (1982). *An analysis of hospital expenditures in Canada* (SC publication No. 83-522E). Ottawa, Ontario, Canada: Department of Supply and Services.

Statistics Canada. (1984). *The elderly in Canada* (SC publication No. 99-932). Ottawa, Ontario, Canada. Department of Supply and Services.

Taylor, M. G. (1978). *Health insurance and Canadian public policy: The seven decisions that created the Canadian health insurance system.* Montreal, Canada: McGill-Queen's University Press.

Taylor, M. G., Stephenson, H. M., & Williams, A. P. (1984). *Medical perspectives on Canadian medicare.* Toronto, Ontario, Canada: York University, Institute for Behaviorial Research.

Taylor, M. G. (1985). The Canadian health system, 1974–1984. In R. G. Evans & G. L. Stoddard (Eds.), *Medicare of maturity: Achievements, lessons and challenges* (pp. 1–30). Toronto, Canada: Irwin Publishing.

Thomas, L. (1983). *The youngest science.* New York: Viking.

6
Geriatric Care: The View from Sweden

Alvar Svanborg

Sweden seems still to be the oldest country in the world as far as the composition of its population is concerned. Approximately 17% of the population is now 65 years old or more, a figure that will increase and reach 18% in 1990. We can also anticipate that in 2025 when the 25-year-olds of 1985 retire—if they at that time also must retire at the age of 65—something between 20% and 23% of the Swedish population will be 65 and above. From certain perspectives, we thus already have experiences with problems of caring for the elderly that other nations will meet in the future.

In this context, I would like to point out that the Scandinavians no longer have the highest longevity. Both males and females in Japan have today the highest longevity in the world (Svanborg et al., 1985). On the other hand, the percentage of elderly in Japan is today considerably lower than that in Sweden, 10% versus 17%.

DIVERSITY OF OLDER POPULATIONS

When we talk about distinctive roles of hospitals for care of the elderly in the future, one obviously central question concerns the possible age–cohort differences among elderly persons and to what extent future cohorts of elderly will need the same quality and quantity of medical service, social support, and care in general as the previous and present generations. I have many times presented our studies of different age cohorts of 70-year-olds in Göteborg, Sweden, but it seems to be reasonable to repeat some of the observations in this context (Rinder et al., 1975; Svanborg, 1977). As far as we can see, the Swedish population in 1985 is manifesting aging and some pathological conditions at chronologically later ages, meaning that older adults keep vitality and good health a little longer today than did the elderly only 10 years ago.

In many national and international contexts these findings in Göteborg have been taken as evidence for a successively lowered need of care of the elderly in the future. I would like to emphasize that we ourselves have never dared to draw that conclusion, namely that the duration of the period of life when we really need medical service and care should become shorter for future elderly than for the elderly of today. Not only in females but in recent years also in males, the future age-specific life expectancy, for example at age 70, is significantly increasing. Although we have the same dream as many others who have been talking about "compression of morbidity and need of care" to a shorter period of life, I would like to emphasize definitely that we have not yet in our studies showed anything except that we seem to postpone the manifestations of aging and the occurrence of definable disorders up to a higher age. But we live, on the other hand, longer. This implies that we have not up to the present time been able to show anything that indicates an ongoing compression of morbidity and need of care in the Swedish population. In planning care for future elderly, it therefore seems to be realistic to plan for the future elderly in the same way as we know that we should have planned for the elderly living today (Svanborg et al., 1982).

EXPLAINING COHORT DIFFERENCES

The basis for these age–cohort differences in the Göteborg population does not seem to be of a genetic nature. During the period studied by us, the migration rate within the population has been low in the Göteborg area. This means that lifestyle and environmental factors apparently play a much more important role, not only for the state of health when we become elderly but also for the rate and manifestations of aging (Svanborg, 1984; Svanborg et al., 1984). One of the consequences of these observations is that we can expect not only positive age–cohort trends but also negative ones. We have lots of indirect evidence that smoking has a negative influence on the density of the skeleton, a phenomenon that is apparently one of the reasons why the incidence of hip fractures is rather dramatically increasing in many areas of Sweden, but not in all (Rundgren et al., 1984). In the year 2000, Göteborg will have at least twice as many hip fractures as could be explained by the aging of the population. The urgent need for preventive measures is illustrated by these figures. The coming generations of females will include much higher percentages of heavy smokers, with all the negative consequences—not only for the overall state of health but also for the rate and manifestations of aging—and will probably need medical service, care, and social support.

LOCATING GERIATRIC CARE

In Sweden, it has been a generally accepted idea that elderly should be allowed to be cared for at home to a greater extent than has previously been common. In some situations this idea has been translated to mean that the elderly need only kindness and care to be allowed to remain at home. Some recent findings from our population illustrate how definitely wrong this interpretation is. In 1984 three fourths of females who died in Sweden were in the age area of 73 or above, and three quarters of the males who died were 67 years old or older. This quartile grouping concerns not only the age of dying, but also the age intervals where the most serious disease occurs. If anybody needs adequate medical resources, it is of course the elderly!

We have in many areas of Sweden a shortage of hospital beds and nursing home beds for the elderly. This is one of the reasons we have organized special hospital-based teams to supplement nursing and rehabilitation facilities. The objective is to improve the possibility for people with long-term illness and need of long-term care to be cared for at home instead of in institutions. We have a feeling that many politicians and organizers of medical care had hoped that a great number of elderly who nowadays are cared for in geriatric hospitals or in nursing homes would have been in such a condition that they could have been allowed to go home and be cared for there instead of in institutions. The organization and the resources for geriatric care is, of course, different in different towns and communities in Sweden. We have, however, made a systematic study of 210 elderly cared for in a "representative" nursing home in the Göteborg area. According to strict medical criteria, approximately one third of these patients might have been treated at home if adequate geriatric nursing facilities could have been offered them in their home situation. And we have thus organized such teams offering really good medical care service at home. Further extensive trials, however, showed that due to social reasons such as the lack of one's own apartment or lack of relatives, 50 out of the 71 patients had to stay in institutional care. I was personally extremely disappointed to find that in spite of all the efforts that we made to find appropriate care facilities for these elderly who might have lived in their own homes, in the end only one institutionalized patient accepted the proposal to move from the safeness of being in a nursing home. I am therefore rather pessimistic about the possibilities for a drastic reduction of the facilities for hospital and nursing home care for elderly in the future, at least in the city of Göteborg. The situation might of course be different in other areas, where there really has been an overproduction of nursing home facilities.

A CONTINUUM OF CARE

When we talk about the need of care and the continuum of care for the elderly, I am eager to emphasize that we should not restrict discussion to the number of hospital beds. We must also emphasize the importance of other features of both hospitals and nursing homes in order to allow us to better cope with the real need of nursing environment of the elderly—and also of younger individuals with chronic disorders. In Göteborg, the main nursing homes are used more or less as a hospital annex of geriatric clinics. This means that we have a possibility for a much better and more dynamic system of geriatric care and rehabilitation. We have, therefore, also been able to use nursing home beds more effectively than would have been possible if the nursing homes had been administered separately. The important role of hospital units and related clinics as a basis for more effective use of both acute hospital beds and long-term care beds has been obvious and will be even more obvious in the future.

TRAINING PERSONNEL

When we talk of a distinctive role of hospitals in the continuum of care for the elderly, we must also point at the qualitative aspects concerning training of personnel. One important area is to widen the knowledge about the physiology of aging versus incidence and prevalence of definable disease in the elderly. Gerontology is really a problem for all medical specialties with the exception of pediatrics and obstetrics. A specialized discipline in medicine should, however, know something distinctive about aging and should have an overview perspective on aging, pathology of the aged, and the different important areas of knowledge concerning need for care. Within medicine geriatricians have to be expected to know more about aging in the elderly than do the other disciplines. Without geriatric units and geriatric clinics within hospitals, as well as close cooperation with the wide sector of long-term care mainly represented by nursing homes, care of the elderly will be no discipline's specialty and will be inadequate and unnecessarily expensive. My final comment therefore is to emphasize that within the framework of hospitals, resources for clinical work, education, and training, as well as research in the fields of medical gerontology and geriatric medicine, are prerequisites for good care of the graying nations (Svanborg, 1983; Svanborg et al., 1984).

REFERENCES

Rinder, L., Roupe, S., Steen, B., & Svanborg, A. (1975). Seventy-year-old people in Gothenburg: A population study in an industrialized Swedish city. I. General presentation of the study. Stencil. *Acta Medica Scandinavica 198,* 397–407.

Rundgren, Å, Eklund, S., & Jonson, R. (1984). Bone mineral content in 70 and 75-year-old men and women: An analysis of some anthropometric background factors. *Age and Ageing, 13,* 6–13.

Svanborg, A. (1977). Seventy-year-old people in Gothenburg: A population study in an industrialized Swedish city. II. General presentation of social and medical conditions. *Acta Medica Scandinavica* (Suppl. 611), 5–37.

Svanborg, A., Landahl, S., & Mellström, D. (1982). Basic issues of health care. In H. Thomae & G. L. Maddox (Eds.), *New perspectives on old age: A message to decision makers. On behalf of the International Association of Gerontology* (pp. 31–52). New York: Springer Publishing Company.

Svanborg, A. (1983). The physiology of ageing in man—diagnostic and therapeutic aspects. In F. I. Caird & J. Grimley Evans (Eds.), *Advanced geriatric medicine 3* (pp. 175–182). London: Pitman.

Svanborg, A. (1984). Ecology, aging and health in a medical perspective. Lecture at the NATO Symposium "Aging and Technological Advances," August 22–26, 1983. In P. K. Robinson, J. Livingstone, & J. Birren (Eds.), *Aging and technological advances* (pp. 159–168). New York: NATO Conference Series, Plenum Press.

Svanborg, A., Berg, S., Nilsson, L., & Persson, G. (1984). A cohort comparison of functional ability and mental disorders in two representative samples of 70-year-olds. In J. Wertheimer & M. Marois (Eds.), *Modern aging research Vol. 5. Senile dementia: Outlook for the future* (pp. 405–409). New York: Alan R. Liss.

Svanborg, A., Shibata, H., Hatano, S., & Matsuzaki, T. (1985). Comparison of ecology, ageing and state of health in Japan and Sweden, the present and previous leaders in longevity. *Acta Medica Scandinavica, 218,* 5–17.

7
Nursing and Care of the Elderly: A View from Israel

Miriam J. Hirschfeld

My view is that of a nurse involved in the various facets of geriatric care: long-term care policy, clinical practice and research, and education. It is a view formed in the reality of Israel, a small country with a rapidly growing aged population. In Israel the old-old (persons 75 and older) represented 28.6% of the aged in 1950, 31.1% in 1980, and are expected to comprise 40.1% of the elderly by 1990. While only 28,000 people (or 3.8% of the population) were age 65 and over when Israel regained statehood in 1948, this number has increased twelvefold to some 340,000 aged and the percentage to 9.8% in the 35 years since statehood (Brookdale Chartbook, 1982; see also Habib & Factor, 1984).

THE EPIDEMIOLOGY OF AN AGING POPULATION

Within less than a generation, demographic and morbidity patterns have changed from those typical of a developing country to those typical of a developed country. While infectious diseases and malnutrition were rampant with the great immigration waves of the early 1950s, these disease patterns have vanished. In their place, chronic illnesses such as cardiovascular disease, cancer, and cerebrovascular diseases have become the major causes of mortality. Forty-five percent of the 350,000 aged (65+) insured in 1984 by Israel's major HMO, Kupat Holim Clalit, received medications for chronic illnesses on a long-term basis.

The demographic and epidemiological changes just described have occured in a country with time-honored respect for the aged. Jews, Moslems, and Christians alike have old traditions holding the elderly in esteem. Israel is also a country with an ideology of egalitarian, universalistic health care, but at the same time, it finds itself in the throes of a severe economic crisis.

AN IMPENDING CRISIS

From my view of aged care, the hospital seems placed in the eye of a storm raging between Scylla and Charybdis. And while this imagery seems exaggerated, I am afraid it is not. The storm itself is the acuteness of the economic crisis with a huge budget deficit that must be covered at close to any cost. The most conspicuous focus of health care, the one where expenditures are highest and most visible, is the hospital; the target group that has the most conspicuous use of this service is the elderly. Those persons 65 and over account for 30% of all bed days in acute care hospitals. They have an annual hospital admission rate per thousand more than double that for the nonelderly. The average duration of hospital stay for the aged is twice as high as that for younger people; 40% to 60% of most hospital departments are occupied by those 65 and over (Brookdale Chartbook, 1982; see also Bergman, 1980).

FINANCING CARE

The financial responsibility for care of the aged in Israel is divided among several agencies. For those insured by Kupat Holim Clalit (Health Insurance Institute of the General Federation of Labour, which insures about 80% of the Israeli population in general and over 90% of the aged population), benefits cover general hospital, community primary care, and rehabilitation services. Payment for long-term care is divided among the individuals and their families, Kupat Holim, and the Ministry of Health, depending on the family's financial status.

Thus, when recently the government insisted that Kupat Holim reduce if not eliminate its huge budget deficit (figures range between $60 million and $400 million, depending on the source of the estimates) the over 1 million hospital bed days used by old people per year figured prominently in the arguments. The problem was intensified because Kupat Holim must find a way to pay for over 1 million bed days of its members in government hospitals. And to further illustrate the atmosphere in which discussions of the role of the hospital in the care of the elderly must be viewed in Israel, the alternatives for reducing costs discussed include dismissing employees, not covering drug expenditures, or discontinuing other essential services such as psychiatric care. In a country where both health care and employment are seen as basic human rights, none of these alternatives are socially acceptable.

On the one hand hospital care for older adults is viewed not only as excessive and overly expensive but also as needless and expendable. On the other hand, hospital care for the sick elderly may be overused because of the lack of adequate community services and insufficient response to the specific needs of old people in a timely way. The inadequacy of response seems due to ageism and therapeutic nihilism (see Chapter 3) and also results from the lack of knowledge among providers of care (see Chapter 4). Old people in hospitals are frequently very impaired and commonly present a syndrome of acute disease. The ominous dyad of confusion and reduced functional ability is common. Confused old persons wetting the bed or crawling into the hospital bed of another patient are so easily labeled senile or demented. What should be seen as an acute reversible state, because so often it is due to exacerbation of multiple chronic diseases and the interaction of multiple drug therapy, turns into a case of "bed-blocking" (Bendel, 1985).

A DISTINCTIVE ROLE FOR HOSPITALS

What then is the role of the hospital in the eye of the storm of economic crisis? In the best interest of the elderly, can we discard hospitals as unresponsive to their needs and therefore expendable? Can we argue that they are too expensive and hence not justified as essential in responding to health care needs of old people? Kane and Vladeck (Chapters 2 and 3) earlier in this book both made a strong point that there is no reason to continue the myth that there are no alternatives to the hospital. On the other hand, there is general agreement that our societies may not have a better alternative to which to turn in securing appropriate care of the elderly. If hospitals are abandoned, the baby may be poured out with the bathwater.

I would like to make the case that the hospital has, in fact, a very important role as *one* link within a health care system designed to promote optimal well-being for the elderly. What is this distinctive role of the hospital? In my view there are two distinctive areas in which hospitals seem to be better equipped than any other entity: acute and emergency care and medical problems where highly specialized services (knowledge and high technology) are needed.

The majority of old people's health problems might be met best by adequately prepared primary health care teams. And a well-developed network of community services has the potential to greatly improve quality of life in old age. Many problems will not demand hospital attention. But the hospital does provide an environment for the most rapid, efficient, and competent assessment and treatment of acute health problems and those problems resulting from exacerbations of chronic diseases. A broken femur, intracranial hemorrhage, the complications faced by an old person who suffers from heart and lung diseases combined with diabetes and high blood pressure, or the trials of living with Parkinson's disease and becoming acutely confused under oncological treatment—these are examples of situations where competent hospital care seems vital.

The role of the hospital for our aged population in Israel therefore remains at the epicenter of intense conflicting pressures.

While rapid demographic and morbidity changes have created an aging population in dire need of the services of the hospital, economic considerations press toward reducing hospital bed days for the elderly. Additional forces are constituted by the prevailing public and professional expectations of modern medicine. Highly sophisticated, high-technology care seems a basic right for everyone, regardless of age. Israel is one of the very few countries, for example, to provide hemodialysis to everyone needing it. Nothing should be too expensive for an individual's health, and economic concerns seem to be unacceptable when weighed against the saving of a human life. This holds particularly true for high-technology emergency care. In conflict with this attitude is the fact that in Israel, as in so many other countries, hospitals have not served our aged population very well. Ageism, therapeutic nihilism, and lack of adequate preparation and knowledge in geriatric care have made hospitals a less than optimal choice for many old persons whose functional ability and self-respect were severely taxed by hospital stays.

ESSENTIAL CHANGES

Essential changes are needed if the hospital is to fulfill its distinctive role within economic reason in the best interest of the elderly. Three of these changes warrant comment:

1. A change in knowledge and attitudes.
2. A change in emphasis within the health care team, from a physician/medicine leadership to a shared responsibility of the health care team (as Williamson advocates) and a decisive role for nursing.
3. A change in the structure of the health care system.

1. *Knowledge and attitudes.* The need for better understanding of human aging has been most eloquently addressed in the previous chapters of this book. There is a need for hospital-based centers of excellence to develop high-level clinical skills and to promote geriatric research, consultation, and teaching. A plan for

changing knowledge and attitudes about the care of the aged is beyond the scope of this discussion, but I should like to mention the vicious cycle of negative attitudes leading to deficient professional education and lack of knowledge, which leads to inadequate care and negative results, thus in turn reinforcing negative attitudes. This cycle can be reversed by sound educational and research efforts leading to quality intervention, which would then lead to positive patient results, thus creating knowledge and reversing negative attitudes in turn (Hirschfeld, 1984; WHO, 1980).

2. *Professional responsibility and leadership.* Although medicine's foremost tasks are diagnosis and treatment, nursing's major task is the management of symptoms and functional disability, as well as the promotion of self-care. Promoting optimal quality of life and functioning not only for the impaired old person but also for the patient's family are major goals for nursing. Traditionally, health care did not cope well with problems of prevention, chronic disease, and handicap. Nursing, following the tradition of medicine, used to focus upon acute and individual interventions. This is an area where change is necessary.

Efforts need to be directed increasingly toward the entire health care spectrum, from preventive care and health maintenance of the well elderly to states of severe dependency among the sick elderly. In addition, the focus must shift from individual care alone to care of the family and to community and environmental interventions. Promotion and teaching of self-care on all these levels will have to be initiated in the hospital if we want to reduce frequent readmissions of the elderly (Hirschfeld, 1985).

A crucial issue relates to the professional competencies we value. The *cure* function usually associated with medicine is valued higher than the *care* function associated with nursing. However, these values only partially correspond to the competencies most strongly effecting the good of the frail and elderly (Jameton, 1984). Especially in hospitals, nursing will have to learn to give priority to caring and tending skills that promote independence and the old person's self-respect. Skills needed in high technology and in emergency care will only be able to benefit old people in hospitals if the "human" nursing skills are effective. Only then will old persons in the "zone of severely reduced reserves"—confused and dependent—be able to preserve their self-respect and benefit from the tremendous achievements of modern medicine.

3. *The structural organization of the health care system.* Before addressing the issue of change in the structure of the health care system, I would like to stress that a basic philosophy underlies all social and health care policy. Kupat Holim's basic principles, which represent Israel's prevailing philosophy of health care, seem worth mentioning:

1. Equality: accessible health care to all
2. Comprehensiveness: health care (physical-mental-social) throughout the life cycle
3. To each according to his needs, regardless of ability to pay

Operationalizing this philosophy leads to the following implications for the organization of services:

1. Services to the aged are an integral part of general health care. Age-segregated services are both inadequate for answering the needs of the elderly, as well as being inefficient economically. Taylor's presentation of Canada's health care system (Chapter 5) gives ample evidence on this point.
2. Because the vast majority of the elderly live in the community, and their health problems are primarily of a chronic nature and of maintaining functional capacity and self-care, the responsibility for this care is centered in the primary community clinic. In Israel these clinics are staffed by nurse–physician primary-care teams. Thirteen hundred such Kupat Holim clinics exist in every urban neighborhood and rural settlement. Nurse-staffed clinics exist in many developing countries that will have to face the challenge of a growing elderly population in the near future. The Alma Ata goal of WHO—"Health for all by the year 2000"— would demand such a development of primary health care. Adequately prepared nurses could take on the responsibility for the care of the elderly in addition to their traditional mother–child care and public health responsibilities.
3. The primary care team has a wide range of back-up services

at its disposal: personal care and homemaker services, rehabilitation, laboratory, day care, family-relief services, and specialist consultation (Factor & Habib, 1984; Factor et al., 1984).

4. The hospital serves as an important back-up service in the areas of acute and emergency care, as well as in those areas where highly specialized knowledge and/or technology are needed. The hospital may also serve as a place to die for those who want aggressive medical care until the end, or those who are unwilling or unable to accept home or hospice death.
5. Care for the aged is multidirectional: from home to community to hospital to long-term care institutions, and back to the home according to changing needs of the old person and the family.
6. Ready availability: Community services must be available around the clock—including weekends and holidays—and geographic spread must be adequate.
7. Health and social services are integrated.
8. Mental health and psychiatric services are an integral part of the general health services.
9. Services to family caregivers are readily available.

For those countries where the infrastructure of a primary community care system exists, as is the case in quite a few of the developing countries, this alternative to a traditional medical model of care seems feasible. A demonstration project aimed at proving the effectiveness of such comprehensive nursing care in the community (with hospital back-up) is now in its planning stages in Graz, Austria, a highly developed urban setting (WHO, 1985).

I do believe that such comprehensive geriatric care has promise to reduce health expenditures while providing quality services to the aged, maintaining independent functioning where possible, and managing dependence when unavoidable. A distinctive role of the hospital is confirmed in those areas where its contribution is unique and most needed: that is, in "high-knowledge," acute emergency care, and in setting the stage for self-care when chronically ill aged become hospitalized.

REFERENCES

Bendel, J. P. (1985). *Bed-blocking in general hospitals by elderly patients waiting for post-discharge arrangements.* Jerusalem: Joint (JDC) Israel Brookdale Institute of Gerontology and Adult Human Development in Israel, R-29-85.

Bergman, S. (1980). *Hospitalization of the elderly: Israel.* Jerusalem: Joint (JDC) Israel Brookdale Institute of Gerontology and Adult Human Development in Israel, R-15-80.

Brookdale Chartbook. (1982). *Aging in Israel.* Jerusalem: Joint (JDC) Israel Brookdale Institute of Gerontology and Adult Development in Israel.

Factor, H., Guttman, M., & Shmueli, A. (1984). *Mapping of the long-term care system for the aged in Israel.* Jerusalem: Joint (JDC) Israel Brookdale Institute of Gerontology and Adult Human Development in Israel, ES-1-84.

Factor, H., & Habib, J. (1984). *The role of institutional and community services in meeting the long-term care needs of the elderly in Israel: The decade of the '80s.* Jerusalem: Joint (JDC) Israel Brookdale Institute of Gerontology and Adult Development in Israel, D-107-84.

Habib, J., & Factor, H. (1984). *The elderly in Israel.* Jerusalem: Joint (JDC) Israel Brookdale Institute of Gerontology and Adult Human Development in Israel. S-20-84.

Grimley Evans, J. (1984). Prevention of age-associated loss of autonomy: Epidemiological approaches. *Journal of Chronic Diseases, 34,* 353–363.

Hirschfeld, M. J. (1984). Ideology, change and aging education. *Gerontology and Geriatrics Education, 4*(3), 3–14.

Hirschfeld, M. J. (1985). Self-care potential: Is it present? *Journal of Gerontological Nursing, 11*(8), 28–34.

Jameton, A. (1984). *Nursing practice, the ethical issues.* Englewood Cliffs, NJ: Prentice Hall.

World Health Organization. (1980, February). *Health care of the elderly: Implications for education and training of physicians and other health professionals.* Discussion paper by A. Svanborg & J. Williamson (WHO EUR/HCE/10/1).

World Health Organization. (1985). *Pilotkprojekt: Pflegerische Grundversorgung von Patienten im eigenen Wohnbereich* (unpublished document, ICP/HSR 301 s04). Graz, Austria.

8

Hospitals and Geriatric Care: A Historical Perspective on Leadership in Health Care

Stanley J. Brody

To ascribe a role in geriatric care to hospitals requires a definition of that type of care, as well as an appreciation of the health care system. In this context it is well to recall that medical care as distinct from health care has been guided by the *Flexner Report* (Flexner, 1960). The primacy of scientific medicine was the message of that report for practice as well as for education and research. In practice, the report established the framework for developing acute-care medicine and defined the role of the aseptic, rational, biomedical research-driven general hospital.

A HISTORICAL PERSPECTIVE

The effect of the *Flexner Report* did not completely take hold until 30 years had elapsed. With the development of antibiotics in the late 1930s, education for medicine became firmly ensconced in academia, and practice was centralized in hospitals; biomedical acute care became dominant. Subsequent to World War II, with significant federal Hill-Burton support, hospitals expanded in numbers of beds and intensity of acute-care service.

In the early 1950s, yet another report was recorded, that of the Commission on Chronic Illness (1957). Studies by this group pointed out that the health problems of the second half of the 20th century would be those of chronic illness, which required a different organization of practice from that focused only on acute care. The then-Surgeon General Leroy Burney called for a progressive series of services: "intensive care, intermediate care, self-care, long-term care, home and ambulatory care"—all programs to be linked on a campus surrounding the hospital (Burney, 1958).

The 1965 enactment of Medicare, in response to the acute care needs of a new, large older population, reinforced the focus of the hospital on the practice of acute care scientific medicine. By 1985, in part as the result of making hospital-based high-tech medicine available to the elderly, life expectancy at age 65 years increased by 20%, bringing about the second demographic revolution of the aged—that of the rapid increase in those over 85 years of age. With this development came an even greater need to augment acute care with the other kinds of service, as suggested by the Chronic Care Commission some 30 years ago.

These are the services Dr. Williamson (Chapter 4) refers to as the continuum. In this country we initially labeled this spectrum of biopsychosocial-oriented services as *comprehensive care* (Brody, 1973). One of the by-products of developing the broad array of comprehensive services was their differentiation into acute and long-term care; into institutional, community, and in-home services; and into medical and health/social services (Brody, 1979). Recently, long-term services have been differentiated between short-term long-term care (STLTC), that is, those services provided within 90 days of hospital discharge whose purpose is to help elderly disabled patients to make the transition to community living, and long-term long-term care (LTLTC), that is, those services required over time to rehabilitate, improve, maintain, and support the chronically disabled. Although both subsets of service involve medical and psychosocial services, STLTC is more medically oriented, whereas LTLTC is psychosocially focused (Brody & Magel, 1987).

Bruce Vladeck (Chapter 3) points out that a key issue in ensuring the appropriate use from among this array of services is one of management. In effect, continuity of care, which is the overriding need of the chronically disabled, can only be achieved through effective management of the service continuum.

Many of the array of services, as Dr. Kane reports (Chapter 2), are psychosocial in nature and reflect a focus on the functional deficits of the older patient as well as on the physical condition. What has not been emphasized enough is that the elderly population we serve is a continually changing, heterogeneous group who seem to be staying healthy as they are becoming older. In that respect, it is important to note what Dr. Burney emphasized over 30 years ago, and what Dr. Williamson reports as an integral part of British geriatric practice: The necessity for rehabilitation is an ever-present part of the continuity of care, providing a climate of therapeutic optimism in the treatment of the elderly (Williams, 1986).

THE CHANGING ROLE OF HOSPITALS

The hospital is part of the continuum. Its role is defined by the services it provides and the management task it undertakes. The hospital is ubiquitous geographically and serves at least half of the elderly population annually on an inpatient or outpatient basis. Both Drs. Kane and Vladeck point out that as the result of many factors, of which prospective payment is a major one, many hospitals are broadening their focus from acute care to include many of the short-term long-term services. In the past 5 years, the number of hospitals providing direct home health care service has increased from 300 to almost 2000. At the same time, hospital provision of nursing home-type beds has likewise increased to 1200. Rehabilitation inpatient and outpatient services have similarly expanded (Hospital Research and Educational Trust, 1986).

The management of hospitals has not changed as precipitously as has their diversity of services. Many hospitals have increased the number and range of services, but it is in no sense a universal response to the awareness of a change in mission. Some hospitals have moved to a new role as a participant in the continuity of care, and a few have assumed a leading role as the manager of such a system. Twenty-five of these institutions are beneficiaries of the Robert Wood Johnson Foundation program Hospital Initiatives in Long-Term Care. Others have developed their own initiatives. The awareness of the importance of the elderly as a "lucrative market" and as a necessary one is gaining credence. Just as for schools of public health, research institutes, and other social agencies, fiscal viability and lucrative markets are meaningful incentives for hospitals. In short, the voluntary sector must market its services.

Some professionals and nonprofit organizations are uncomfortable with the use of the word *marketing* in connection with their activities, incorrectly identifying it with selling and exploitation. To quote the author of the major book on the subject: "A *societal marketing orientation* holds that the main task of the organization is to determine the needs, wants, and interest of the target markets and to adapt the organization to delivering satisfaction that preserve or enhance the consumers' and society's well being" (Kotler, 1975). The earning of profit from or the underwriting of the costs of services created by such marketing should not be seen in negative terms only.

POSITIVE ASPECTS OF MARKETING

Marketing in no way compromises the values on which voluntary activities are based—values in which it justifiably takes pride. To the contrary, it is precisely those values that must be marketed—that is, the commitment to quality services and facilities that attend to the quality of life. On the other hand, as we have pointed out, this response is not unique to hospitals. Accordingly, leadership in the development and management of continuity of care could be assumed by HMOs, SNFs, physician groups, or foreign corporations, dependent on individual enterprise and the ecology of place. On balance, however, as Kane and Vladeck agree, the hospital is a logical source of such management because of experience and resources.

Some of the problems hospitals have in assuming the role of leadership in providing and managing continuity of services for the geriatric patient are the result of the training and experience of administrators and providers, which have been oriented to acute care. The rewards of the Medicare system are in terms of acute care, while there is an absence of public support for a broad continuum of services as well as for case management. The award system in education remains high-tech, biomedically oriented, whether measured in terms of NIH grants, educational advancement, medical status, or scientific awards. All providers and most administrators have interned in high-tech settings. Patients themselves demand scientific medicine and resist any awareness of the possibility of disability. Disability is expectable but never expected by aging families, so that planning and the financing of support services have few advocates among elderly consumers. As Engel (1977, p. 130) observed, "the biomedical model has . . . become a cultural imperative . . . it has now acquired the status of *dogma.*" In other words, scientific medicine is the witchcraft of Western civilization.

On the other hand, the new prospective payment system encourages the development of STLTC services and the reallocation of acute care resources to step-down services. Hospitals are slowly undertaking educational programs to advise their boards, administrators, staff, and physicians regarding the new needs of their elderly patients for continuity of care. The dynamic scope of hospital services is testament to change under way.

AN OPEN MARKET FOR LEADERSHIP

In summary, I agree with Dr. Kane that there is an open market for leadership and that the hospital must aggressively market a broader range of service to its elderly consumers if it is to be a leader and not a follower. It must be reemphasized that the most difficult task of marketing is that of convincing the older consumers of their need for continuity of care. Until private or public third-party funds are available, changing the role of the hospital will continue to be a difficult task; and those funds will not become available until the attitude of the elderly consumer changes.

I agree, too, with Dr. Vladeck when he asserts that hospitals present the best opportunity for leadership. Their capital-rich position, management experience, multidisciplinary staffs, and funnel position in servicing the aged all reinforce this position.

Dr. Williamson's success leaves little room for disagreement. Case management is the way to manage continuity of care. It must be noted that, from the results of the Robert Wood Johnson Foundation experience and other research, a minority of the elderly will need such services. A Delphic-based survey suggests that perhaps between 10% and 18% of Medicare admissions to hospitals may need such assistance.

And finally, Dr. Taylor's conclusion, that the issue is more political than it is provider- or data-responsive, is overriding. In the last analysis, it remains a value issue for the electorate to decide—just as they did with Social Security and Medicare—whether continuity of care is their critical need.

REFERENCES

Brody, S. J. (1973). Comprehensive health care for the elderly: An analysis. *Gerontologist, 13*(4), 412–418.

Brody, S. J. (1979). The thirty-to-one paradox: Health needs and medical solutions. *National Journal, 11*(44), 1869–1873.

Brody, S. J., & Magel, J. S. (1985). Step-down care promotes vertical integration. *Hospitals, 59*(23), 76–77.

Brody, S. J., & Magel, J. S. (1987). LTC: The long and short of it. In C. Eisdorfer (Ed.), *Reshaping health care for the elderly: Recommendations for national policy.*

Burney, L. E. (1958). Health and hospitals for an aging population. *Transactions and Studies of the College of Physicians of Philadelphia, 26*(2), 59–70.

Commission on Chronic Illness. (1957). *Chronic illness in a large city.* Cambridge, MA: Harvard University Press.

Engel, G. L. (1977). The need for a new medical model: A challenge for biomedicine. *Science, 196*(4286), 129–136.

Flexner, A. (1960). *Medical education in the United States and Canada.* Washington, DC: Science and Health Publications. (Commissioned in 1910 by the Carnegie Foundation for the Advancement of Teaching)

Hospital Research and Educational Trust. (1986). *Emerging trends in aging and long-term care services.* Chicago: Author.

Kotler, P. (1975). *Marketing for non-profit organizations* (2nd ed.). Englewood Cliffs, NJ: Prentice-Hall.

Williams, T. F. (1986). The aging process: Biological and psychosocial considerations. In S. J. Brody & G. E. Ruff (Eds.), *Aging and rehabilitation: Advances in the state of the art.* New York: Springer Publishing Company.

9
Transforming the American Hospital

Mathy Mezey

There is no question that we are witnessing a transformation of the American hospital (Stevens, 1986). The hospital as we know it today will have changed dramatically over the next 10 years. Although there are multiple, complex factors contributing to these changes, the driving force is the demand for health care services by an ever-increasing pool of elderly, chronically ill patients. We are only now beginning to understand that acute diseases that afflict younger adults and the well elderly for the most part require only intermittent attention and in many instances are best managed in day surgery units or short-term admissions, followed by recuperation at home. On the other hand, chronic illnesses that are not amenable to cure but are highly responsive to care require sustained attention, because symptoms wax and wane over the course of a person's life (Strauss, 1975). Rabkin (1986) has suggested that future hospitals will resemble a two-tiered wedding cake, with a small layer symbolizing intensive-care units sitting atop a much larger base that resembles an old-age home.

OPTIONS FOR HOSPITALS

Hospitals have several options for how to respond to these changes in service demands, all of which carry certain risks. First, they can choose to ignore such changes and to continue with business as usual—cutting services, closing beds, and diminishing the nursing staff in order to maintain financial solvency. Such diminished facilities may, however, fail to capture a sufficient market share to remain in existence. Second, hospitals can choose to concentrate on the upper tier of the cake, offering only highly technological care and establishing themselves as specialized tertiary care centers. Such institutions, however, are highly vulnerable to future technological advances that may render current practices obsolete.

A third strategy, which appears to appeal to the majority of hospitals, is to restructure services and practice to be more responsive to the needs of patients with chronic illness. This strategy requires hospitals to come to grips with the difference between the care of patients with chronic illnesses and those with acute illnesses.

COMPLEMENTARY SERVICES

These changes within hospitals are occurring at the same time that there has been a reassessment of the customary division of services among acute care hospitals, nursing homes, and home care agencies and the development by nursing homes of discharge planning modules and home care services. Fundamental to a rational reordering of care for the chronically ill elderly is this recognition of the interdependence of the elements that comprise the system. Hospitals, nursing homes, and home care agencies can profitably cooperate to improve access to care, assure appropriate levels of care, influence reimbursement policy, and rectify existing or impending gaps in care (Mezey & Lynaugh, 1982).

While offering complementary services, hospitals should not and do not provide the same services as do nursing homes and home care agencies. Hospitals provide a unique and distinctive complex of services: diagnosis and management of acute illness and trauma; management of exacerbations of chronic illness; and "bridge" units/services to correctly identify and prepare patients for home care or nursing home care (geriatric assessment and rehabilitation).

Nursing homes, too, offer unique health care services. In fact there is no alternative to nursing home care, just as there is no alternative to care in intensive care units or in coronary care units, when patients are appropriately placed in these facilities. Nor do nursing homes and home care agencies usually offer duplicative services. For example, nursing homes are much more likely to care for cognitively impaired patients with urinary incontinence than are home care agencies (Weissert, 1985).

It is precisely because of the different roles of hospitals, nursing homes, and home care agencies and their dependence on each other to provide a full range of services that hospitals can no longer remain aloof as to the quality of care provided in nursing homes and by home care agencies. Rather, hospitals now have major incentives to involve themselves in assuring adequate standards of care across the continuum of services in the health care system.

Although the roles of hospitals, nursing homes, and home care agencies are different and distinct, the patients in these facilities are similar and overlapping (i.e., primarily older and presenting with or having multiple, concomitant, chronic illnesses). These patients have as their primary goal the drive to maintain, regain, or attain the greatest possible degree of independence. The challenge to hospitals is to administer acute care services efficiently so that they only minimally delay, undermine, or interfere with the patient's resumption of function and ongoing management of their health problems. To meet this challenge requires development of new geriatric services with special attention to the collaborative relationship of medicine and nursing.

FUNCTIONAL AND REHABILITATIVE OUTCOMES

Acute-care hospitals will need to shift their focus from that of medical diagnosis and treatment to consideration of functional and rehabilitative outcomes. Physicians must not only diagnose and manage illnesses, but must also collaborate with others to assure that adequate attention is paid to rehabilitation and functional goals. Nurses, on the other hand, have traditionally concerned themselves with the patient's care. According to Henderson (1966):

> The unique function of the nurse is to assist the individual, sick or well, in the performance of those activities contributing to health or its recovery (or to peaceful death) that he would perform unaided if he had the necessary strength, will or knowledge. And to do this in such a way as to help him gain independence as rapidly as possible. (p. 15)

Nurses then are the linchpin in the patient's recovery process, and they need the necessary knowledge and authority to adjust the plan of care for older persons to accommodate individual needs and to assure adequate recovery. Rabkin (1986) sees the hospital as:

> a place of 24-hour highly professionalized nursing care in which periodic perturbations are generated by physicians.

In an attempt to identify appropriate models of care for elderly patients, it is not surprising that hospitals have turned to nursing homes, in which nursing staffs have a long history of providing care for older, chronically ill patients. Sixty-six percent of nursing home patients need help with personal care (i.e., bathing, feeding, toileting); 66% of nursing home patients have two or more chronic illnesses (Mezey & Lynaugh, 1982).

INNOVATIVE SERVICES

Practices common to nursing homes are now being tested in acute care facilities. Unneeded acute care beds have been converted into hospital-based long term care units and swing beds. Such units provide ongoing supportive and rehabilitative services, once the acute care needs of patients have been satisfied (Brody & Persil, 1984). Several hospitals have developed cooperative care programs, where families are invited to live in the hospital and to participate in the patient's care in preparation for discharge (Rosa & Mulcahy, 1980). In other instances, hospital units have been restructured to promote early independence and to reinforce positive expectations for recovery. Such units encourage early ambulation, the use of personal clothing, communal dining, and the deployment of rehabilitation resources on patient units (Boyer et al., 1986), all common practices in nursing homes. Other hospitals are suggesting lend/lease programs, whereby hospital staff spend time in nursing homes learning to care for chronically disabled elderly (Robert Wood Johnson Foundation Teaching Nursing Home Program, 1986).

PERSONNEL DEVELOPMENT IN GERIATRIC NURSING

Hospitals need to take several steps to assure the availability of resources and personnel necessary to achieve geriatric goals. First, strong interdisciplinary geriatric linkages are needed to provide planning, delivery, and evaluation of geriatric services across professions (e.g., medicine, nursing, social work). Second, intradisciplinary strategies for delivery of services need to be established. Nursing departments need a structure for service delivery that includes the development of a geriatric department or committee, the availability of geriatric nurse specialists, an educational plan for nursing personnel, and mechanisms for discharge planning and collaborative relationships with nursing homes and with home care agencies.

Adequate numbers of master's level geriatric nurse specialists are needed to provide direct patient care, conduct staff education, and formulate interdisciplinary policies and practice. It has been recommended that large hospitals maintain a ratio of 3 nurse specialists per 100 beds, and that smaller hospitals maintain a ratio of 2 per 100 beds (*Nursing Personnel,* 1986). There is no question that geriatric nurse specialists should be adequately represented in this specialist group. Geriatric nurse practitioners (GNPs), because of their proven skills in clinical decision making and management, coupled with experience in working with physicians, are ideal nursing providers in acute care settings. GNPs have served on interdisciplinary geriatric assessment teams and are effective in increasing staff knowledge of geriatric nursing practice (Sullivan, 1986).

The informal bedside teaching, rounds, and in-service education that emanates from implementing geriatric services is considerably strengthened when geriatric nurse specialists have faculty appointments in schools of nursing. The experience of the Robert Wood Johnson Foundation Teaching Nursing Home Program (Aiken et al., 1985; Mezey et al., 1985) suggests that such collaboration strengthens both the clinical practice and the educational programs. The clinical site has access to resources in the school that enhance practice and promote research. The school enlarges its pool of clinically competent faculty who, by serving as role models, are excellent resources for recruiting students and new practitioners into careers in geriatric nursing.

REFERENCES

Aiken, L., Mezey, M., Lynaugh, J., & Buck, C. (1985). Sicker patients and constrained resources: An impending crisis in nursing homes. *Journal of the American Geriatrics Association, 33,* 3.

Boyer, N., Christy Chuang, J., & Gipper, D. (1986). An acute care geriatric unit. *Nursing Management, 17,* 5.

Brody, S., & Persil, N. (1984). *Hospitals and the aged—The new world market.* Radcliffe, MO: Aspen Publications.

Henderson, V. (1966). *The nature of nursing.* New York: Macmillan.

Mezey, M., & Lynaugh, J. (1982). *Imperatives for long term care.* Position paper prepared for National Commission on Nursing, Chicago, IL.

Mezey, M., Lynaugh, J., & Aiken, L. (1985). The Robert Wood Johnson Foundation Teaching Nursing Home Program. In E. Schneider (Ed.), *The teaching nursing home: A new approach to geriatric research, education and clinical care.* Washington, DC: National Institute on Aging (NIH).

Nursing Personnel: Continuing Education. Planning for needs and resources in the Mid-Atlantic Region. (1986, June). Preliminary report, Middle Atlantic Region Nurses Association (MARNA), Teachers College, Columbia University.

Rabkin, M., (1986, April). *The sociology of the hospital.* Paper presented at The

Future of the Hospital, conference sponsored by the United Hospital Fund of New York, Philadelphia.

Robert Wood Johnson Foundation Teaching Nursing Home Program at Georgetown University and Greater Southeastern Hospital Center. (1986). Personal communication.

Rosa, N., & Mulcahy, N. (1980). An adventure in geriatric nursing. *Journal of Gerontological Nursing, 6,* 8.

Stevens, R. (1986). The changing hospital. In L. Aiken & D. Mechanic (Eds.), *Application of social science to clinical medicine and health policy.* New Brunswick, NJ: Rutgers University Press.

Strauss, A. (1975). *Chronic illness and the quality of life.* St. Louis: Mosby.

Sullivan, E. (1986). Tertiary care centers: A role for the geriatric nurse clinician. *Oasis, 3,* 1.

Weissart, W. (1985). Seven reasons why it is so difficult to make community-based LTC cost-effective. *Health Service Research, 20,* 4.

10
The Distinctive Role of the Hospital in the Continuum of Care for the Elderly: A Critical Commentary

Anne R. Somers

The chapters by Kane, Taylor, Vladeck and Williamson in this volume are both interesting and instructive. They provide excellent introductions to health care of the elderly in three major countries—the U.K. (with special emphasis on Scotland), Canada, and the U.S. By focusing on very different aspects of the subject, each author also identifies and discusses major issues facing physicians, hospitals, and other health care providers in these countries. Not surprisingly, the issues they identify vary widely, depending in part on the viewpoint and experience of the author and in part on the political and professional context of the country involved.

POINTS OF VIEW

For example, Dr. Williamson of Edinburgh (Chapter 4), writing from a vantage point of 40 years of national experimentation with geriatric medicine in the United Kingdom, which is longer than in any other country, focuses on the question, "What is the best model for the future development of geriatric medicine?" By implication, this includes the question of what is the best type of hospital geriatric service. Of the four possible options he presents, Dr. Williamson indicates clear preference for a hospital-based selective referral service led by physician specialists in geriatric medicine, assisted by other health professionals, and accepting referrals from community-based GPs. This service works closely with consultants in internal medicine and with other traditional specialists who continue to care for older patients who do not meet the special medical and/or socioeconomic criteria distinguishing the geriatric patient.

By contrast, Dr. Kane (Chapter 2) writes from the viewpoint of the United States, where neither the medical profession, the hospital industry, nor the principal public and private funding agencies have decided whether there is, or should be, a specialty of geriatric medicine, and where the entire health care industry is currently in a state of confusion and transition precipitated by a massive cost-containment movement. He emphasizes the growing battle for turf between hospitals and community agencies over control of long-term care. In this chaotic situation, with institutions changing their definition of mission and function almost overnight in response to financial needs and competitive pressures, Dr. Kane even finds it necessary to ask, "is there such a thing as a hospital?"—a question that must seem a little absurd to the Scots and the Canadians.

Dr. Kane's wry conclusion that "some hospitals may appropriately view an expanded role in long-term care as in their best interest, and some of these may be in areas where such a role represents a benefit to the community" is probably justified in view of many disturbing recent developments in hospital finance, organization, and marketing. But it ignores the fact that we could ask many similar questions with respect to other health care institutions, for example: "What is a home health agency?" "What is an HMO or PPO?" Even, "What is an insurance company?"

Dr. Vladeck (Chapter 3) presents a very different American perspective. He too recognizes the confusion and transitional nature of current health care patterns and relationships. But, unlike Kane, he accepts as both inevitable and desirable the growing interdependence between the hospital and the elderly—albeit with numerous cautions and caveats related primarily to current hospital and financial inadequacies. In his words, "rather than resisting this trend [wherein hospitals seek to become providers of a broader spectrum of geriatric services], advocates of better services for the elderly might do better by seeking to capitalize on it as a vehicle for beginning the massive but essential task of educating hospital managers, physicians, nurses, and other professionals in how to do a better job."

Dr. Taylor (Chapter 5) writes as a Canadian. Unlike the U.K., Canada is not yet committed to a speciality of geriatric medicine and somewhat resembles the U.S. in its many-faceted groping toward a viable pattern of long-term care. But unlike the U.S., Canada has a universal national health insurance program that includes long-term care and provides a basic political consensus and organizational framework within which the new Canadian LTC institutions can develop without having to cannibalize each other. Although not explicitly stated, to me the central issue of the Taylor discussion is whether universal health insurance is a necessary political and financial prerequisite to redefining the distinctive or appropriate role of the hospital in the care of the elderly.

Clearly, we are here privileged to share four excellent presentations with great relevance to the central issue: "What, if anything, is the distinctive role of the hospital in the continuum of health care of the elderly?" At the same time, I am forced to say that none really comes to grips with this central issue. Only Dr. Taylor acknowledges at the outset that he will not attempt to do so.

My own view is, inevitably, that of an American who has long been active in, or associated with, both hospital-based and community-based health care programs. I also speak as an experienced Medicare enrollee and the wife of a seriously disabled 74-year-old long-term care patient with 6 years experience in operating a home care program for him. Throughout this long period, Princeton Hospital has played a major role in our lives—on two occasions life-saving, at other times disappointing, but always central.

DISTINCTIVE ROLES FOR HOSPITALS

It is now possible to identify those roles or functions that are distinctive to the hospital at the present time and those that will or should continue to be distinctive even if we achieve a more rational and efficient system of financing and organizing care in this country.

First, under currently dominant patterns of care, there are four major functions that most elderly patients in the U.S. expect of their hospitals, and which, at the present time, might be considered distinctive if not indispensible:

1. Site of major surgery and intensive care for serious, acute illness
2. Site of 24-hour reliable emergency services
3. Principal site for expensive diagnostic and therapeutic procedures (high technology)
4. Principal site for dying

Obviously, many hospitals are in addition involved in such areas as operation of ambulatory facilities, mental health, rehabilitation, alcoholism, drug abuse, home care, hospice care, other chronic or long-term care facilities or programs, discharge planning, social work, case management, health promotion and patient education, and provision of office space for attending physicians. The American Hospital Association, the Catholic Hospital Association, the New Jersey Hospital Association, as well as many related organizations and individual institutions, are now actively exploring the possibility of hospital expansion into new areas of health care for the elderly (Tedesco, 1985).

I, for one, have generally welcomed the hospital's extension of its traditional acute care role into these newer ends of the health care continuum (Somers, 1971). However, these are functions that can be and, in many instances, are being carried out by other institutions and agencies. Whether they can be carried out more efficiently by a hospital or by a nonhospital body is still a debatable issue that in the present U.S. transitional situation cannot be answered categorically one way or the other. Perhaps in the U.S. it never will be, given our commitment to pluralistic arrangements.

For the purpose of our discussion, however, that is not the issue. The question before us is the *distinctive* role of the hospital. In this context, the four functions I have cited are the principal ones. They constitute an irreducible quartet that must be maintained and adequately funded—if not in the hospital, then in some thoroughly reliable alternate site—if our elderly are not to suffer.

A NEED FOR BALANCE

It may seem to some a bit out of character for one who has so long stressed the need for more preventive and long-term services to emphasize now the acute care function. But what I have always been pleading for is a sense of balance in the allocation of resources—and I still do. While it is clear that we need further significant transfer of resources from acute to chronic care, it is also clear that, in the indiscriminate scramble to cut hospital costs and deinstitutionalize functions and patients, it could end up costing more money in the long run, as it probably did in the analogous case of the policy toward the mentally ill.

There is no question that hospital costs have risen disproportionately during the past quarter of a century. But was this due to the few who were attempting to develop nontraditional functions such as discharge planning, home care, or patient education? Or was this due to the publicly mandated open-ended retroactive cost-based reimbursement system? Again, this is not the topic before us. But in trying to define those services that are *distinctive* to the hospital, it is impossible not to consider factors of appropriateness and efficiency. And my plea is that we not confuse the need for fixed or prospective payment rates for *all* health care providers, including hospitals, with any urge to punish or even isolate the hospital from the rest of the continuum. As usual in such turf battles, it is the patient who suffers most.

One cannot disregard the ominous trend to "bottom-line" health care in the U.S. But this is a trend not confined to hospitals. In fact, traditionally, for-profit enterprise has played a larger role in long-term care than it has in acute care. Nor do I say that the deinstitutionalization of many elderly patients and the "unbundling" of some hospital functions are not both desirable and feasible. But it is my belief that if these goals are to be achieved safely and to the benefit of the patient, they will have to be undertaken much more cautiously and carefully than is often the case at present. I also suspect that the net financial result may often be more, rather than less, expensive. Again, I rule out the distorting influence of the old blank-check reimbursement of hospitals.

EXPLORING ALTERNATIVES

As an illustration, we consider one institution for the elderly that has succeeded in taking over two of the four distinctive hospital functions listed earlier and has done so to the distinct benefit, rather than detriment, of the elderly themselves. I refer to Medford Leas, a Quaker-sponsored nonprofit continuing care retirement community (CCRC) in southern New Jersey. Opened in 1972, Medford Leas was one of the first CCRCs in that part of the country. With approximately 500 residents, it provides independent housing, communal dining, social and recreational activities, essential transportation, and—very importantly—a lifetime contractual guarantee of comprehensive health and medical services (Medford Leas, 1984; Lois E. Forrest, Executive Director, personal communication, 1985, June 26 and July 8).

The health and medical services include a 24-hour residential emergency-call system, primary care (including periodic physicals provided by a full-time medical director and staff), prescription drugs, payment of Medicare deductibles and co-insurance for referred specialty care and hospitalization, home health visits for short-term illness, four levels of long-term care (skilled nursing, intermediate A and B, and residential or personal), and hospice care. Dental and routine eye care are not covered but are available on-site.

To be eligible for payment of Medicare co-insurance, residents must accept the gatekeeper concept and go to physicians designated by the medical director. They must also accept his guidance regarding drugs. The CCRC uses nearby Memorial Hospital of Burlington County for most hospitalizations and several Philadelphia hospitals for specialty care. It has transfer agreements with these hospitals and written contracts with some 100 local and Philadelphia physicians, all of whom have agreed to accept assignment for Medford Leas patients.

As a result of this combination of sheltered living arrangements, easy access to the full continuum of care, and benevolent patient-care management, Medford Leas has become the true center of health care for its residents and has thus altered the role of the hospital in this particular community. Of the four distinctive functions that the hospital has to provide in most communities today, Medford Leas has taken over two: (1) Through its residential surveillance system and its 24-hour skilled-nursing facility (SNF), it provides round-the-clock reliable emergency service that is essential to older people, many of whom live alone. (2) Through its highly skilled nursing facility and hospice-type program, it provides a site of choice for most deaths. Out of 34 deaths that occurred in the past year 27 (about 80%) took place in its SNF, only 2 or 3 in a hospital. Thus it appears that with adequate out-of-hospital facilities, services, and coordinated management, two of the four currently distinctive hospital functions can be provided out-of-hospital without endangering patients. Indeed, considering that the average age of Medford Leas residents at death is 85.4 years, it would appear that they have benefited significantly.

However, it must be noted that these benefits are not cheap. Leaving aside the substantial entry fee and monthly payment that such institutions require, it is useful to compare their medical costs with the national average. Most of the CCRCs attempt to compute their average annual per capita medical costs so that their residents can use this figure for income tax purposes. The Medford Leas figure for 1984 was approximately $7700 (Forrest, 1985). This may be compared with a 1984 projection by the Health Care Financing Administration for the entire elderly population of $4200 (Waldo, 1985).

The two figures in this comparison are not strictly comparable. On the one hand, the CCRC figure is less complete than the national figure because it does not include costs paid by Medicare, the costs of dental care, nonprescription drugs, and a few other noncovered services. On the other hand, the age distribution is quite different. The average age of Medford Leas residents is 82; the median age of the general 65+ population is about 72. The effect of this 10-year differential is evident in the high proportion of Medford Leas health care expenditures going for nursing home care—over 53% compared to a national figure of 21% (Waldo, 1985).

Despite these discrepancies, the Medford Leas figures provide useful cautions to any who may think that nonhospital services are automatically less expensive than hospital services of the same quality and that we can solve the current cost problems in this country primarily through dehospitalization of older patients. To paraphrase Robert Kane's provocative conclusion: Some community agencies or institutions may appropriately view an expanded role in care for the elderly as in their best interest. Some of these may be in areas where such a role also represents a benefit to the patients.

In other words, proceed to dehospitalize with caution. Don't destroy the hospital unless you have something better to put in its place—and then be sure the patient can pay for it!

I conclude with five points.

1. I agree with Bruce Vladeck (Chapter 3) that, in most U.S. communities, "the elderly are now central to the hospital system and hospitals are central to comprehensive care" of the elderly.
2. The precise pattern of relationship between the hospital and other health care institutions caring for the elderly will vary greatly in accordance with our pluralistic society.
3. In any case, the hospital should and will continue to play a

distinctive role with respect to the diagnosis and treatment of serious illness in the elderly.

4. The hospital's future role with respect to the care of chronic and terminal illness remains to be seen and will depend on many factors, including:

    - community attitudes
    - attitude of other providers in the community
    - attitude of the hospital's medical staff
    - the hospital's general acceptance of the newer concepts of geriatric medicine
    - developments in medical education with respect to geriatric medicine; and
    - the adequacy of reimbursement/payment for such services

    There is obviously a hen-and-egg relationship between the financial and professional factors. Without adequate financing, sustained professional interest can never be assured. Without serious professional interest, adequate financing cannot be assured.

5. Finally, it is my enduring conviction that if all elements of the comprehensive care spectrum are to be made available to the elderly patient on an unbiased basis, with both the hospital programs and community-based programs playing their appropriate roles and with effective quality controls, it will only be possible through some form of national health insurance (NHI). I realize that the very term *NHI* is politically unpopular today. But I am sure that we will come back to it—perhaps under some other name and in our own peculiar American fashion—within the decade.

REFERENCES

Medford Leas: A caring community. (1984). Medford, NJ: Author.

Somers, A. R. (1971). Rationalization of community health services and the role of the hospital. In *Health care in transition: Directions for the future* (pp. 99–126). Chicago: Hospital Research and Educational Trust.

Tedesco, J. A. (1985). Elderly require shift in hospital resources. *Hospitals, 59,* 53–63.

Waldo, D. R., & Lazenby, H. C. (1984). Demographic characteristics and health care use and expenditures by the aged in the U.S., 1977–1984. *Health Care Financing Review, 6,* 1–29.

Index